2/11

3000 800065 34919
St. Louis Community College

Queer Questions, Clear Answers

Queer Questions, Clear Answers

The Contemporary Debates
on Sexual Orientation

Thomas S. Serwatka

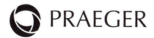 PRAEGER

AN IMPRINT OF ABC-CLIO, LLC
Santa Barbara, California • Denver, Colorado • Oxford, England

Library of Congress Cataloging-in-Publication Data

Serwatka, Thomas S.
    Queer questions, clear answers : the contemporary debates on sexual orientation /
Thomas S. Serwatka.
        p. cm.
    Includes bibliographical references and index.
    ISBN 978-0-313-38612-1 (hard copy : alk. paper) — ISBN 978-0-313-38613-8 (ebook)
1. Sexual orientation.   I. Title.
    HQ23.S457   2010
    306.76—dc22   2010002196

ISBN: 978-0-313-38612-1
EISBN: 978-0-313-38613-8

14   13   12   11   10   1   2   3   4   5

This book is also available on the World Wide Web as an eBook.
Visit www.abc-clio.com for details.

Praeger
An Imprint of ABC-CLIO, LLC

ABC-CLIO, LLC
130 Cremona Drive, P.O. Box 1911
Santa Barbara, California 93116-1911

This book is printed on acid-free paper (∞)

Manufactured in the United States of America

In loving memory of James Austin Owens
February 15, 1952–April 21, 1990
I wish we had had more time to celebrate life together.

Contents

1

Introduction

Over the past several decades, our cultural conversations on homosexuality have dramatically changed. Once a topic for the occasional off-color joke or put down or the relatively obscure movie or theatrical production, homosexuality has moved to center stage in our public discourse—with ongoing debates in media, church pulpits, polling booths, and courtrooms across the country. And with each change in these conversations, the stakes seem to get higher. For some of us, reversing the growing acceptance of the homosexual lifestyle is an absolute imperative if we stand any chance of restoring our disintegrating morals. For others, the shift in attitudes represents remarkable steps toward securing the long-sought freedom to build families with same-sex partners. With the stakes so high, it is predictable, but nonetheless disappointing, that much of our public dialogue has degenerated into little more than sound bites and chatter designed to spin the data so that our truth becomes everyone's truth—those same strategies we use in the worst of our political campaigns.

These sound bites represent recurring themes that deserve to be examined. But more often than not, all we remember is the bravado, failing to look at the accuracy of the underlying data.

Having been victimized by and, I confess, having engaged in these tactics, a few years ago I made a personal decision to step back and carefully consider the often-asked questions about homosexuality. For my own sake I needed to stop and look carefully at what stood behind the bombast on all sides of the arguments. What lessons could I uncover by peering through the lenses of the zoologist and the jurist, the psychologist and the politician, the demographer and the historian, the religious scholar and the geneticist, and the artist and the economist? As a society our conversations may have become little more than rants and raves, but these men and women were putting together a compelling, if still incomplete, picture of homosexuality and its impact on our society, and I wanted to understand that picture. Fortunately, as I worked across these disparate academic disciplines, I was guided by some incredible literary and personal mentors on all sides of the argument.

As I continued my journey, I began to put fingers to keyboard to write this book, in an attempt to share what I had learned in the quest to answer my questions. The text is, as the title states, framed around queer questions: (a) questions that focused on queer people—gay men and lesbians and bisexuals—and (b) questions that are "strange" in their nature or questions designed to put someone at a disadvantage.[1]

> Although the word "queer" has a history of being used as a demeaning or derogatory reference to gay men and lesbians, in the 1980s the term was reclaimed by a group of people who challenged society's sexual and gender norms: gay men, lesbians, transsexuals, transvestites, intersex individuals, and anyone else who fell outside traditional heterosexual patterns. For those among us who reclaimed the word "queer," queerness was to be celebrated, challenging the assumption that heterosexuality should set societal standards. Queer theorists also take issue with often-heard theories presented by other LGBT advocates—for example, that sexual orientation is an innate or essential part of the individual.
>
> Although queer theory is discussed at points in this text, I do not suggest that it is the sole or even best source of the answers to many of the questions asked in these pages. But I do use the word as a celebration of difference and with a sense of open acceptance of homosexuality, bisexuality, and transsexuality.

I drew these queer questions from our contemporary conversations in which gay men, lesbians, bisexuals, transsexuals, and intersex individuals must explain and defend themselves. For example, when asking, "Why do homosexuals have to flaunt their sexual orientation?" few of us ever consider asking what would seem to be the obvious corresponding question:

"Why do heterosexuals have to hold hands or kiss each other in public?" This second question seems unnecessary or irrelevant: Why would we need to explain or justify the natural? It is our reality. For some of the queer questions asked throughout the text, I also point to a corollary or corresponding question—one that is framed from a perspective of the homosexual minority as opposed to the heterosexual majority: "Why am I labeled as a potential child molester when heterosexual men, the group that perpetrates the majority of these crimes, escape this accusation?"

In responding to these questions, I have provided what for me are clear answers—that is, answers that are completely candid, even if that means pointing to the inevitable flaws we might find in some lesbian, gay, or bisexual (LGB) persons or the flaws we might find in those who would oppose lesbian and gay rights. These answers are summarized at the end of each chapter in a section titled Straight Talk.

Of course, this commitment to clear answers and straight talk does not come with a promise of simple or absolute conclusions. In these pages, you won't find definitive statements as to whether there is a gay gene or whether sexual orientation is immutable, nor should you find definitive answers to many of our questions anywhere else. Biology, history, and the social sciences—the fields from which we draw much of the information on the subject of sexual orientation—rarely afford us the luxury of final and irrefutable truths. But we can find some very strong and compelling hypotheses.

THE CHAPTERS AND THE QUESTIONS

Throughout the manuscript we examine a number of queer questions. Eight of these questions and their corollaries and corresponding questions serve as the organizing framework for the next eight chapters of this text.

In chapter 2, we begin by asking what it means to be homosexual or bisexual. Is our sexual orientation defined by physical attraction, sexual behavior, or our self-identity? If I say, "I am absolutely *not* homosexual," but whenever an opportunity arises, I am out sleeping with a member of the same sex, does my disclaimer ring true? If the Catholic priest never engages in sex, can he still be gay? In the second half of the chapter, we move to the question of how many gay men and lesbians there are. Is it 1 percent of the population, the answer offered by some of us who oppose gay and lesbian rights? Is it 10 percent of the population as suggested by several gay and lesbian rights advocates, based on their assumption of what Kinsey said? And what differences does it make whatever the magic number is?

In the third chapter we explore the origins of sexual orientation. Are gay men and lesbians the product of poor parenting or a liberal and permissive society? Is the origin of homosexuality and bisexuality found in our genetics or triggered by some other biological agent? Or is sexual orientation nothing more than a set of labels we apply to people as a mechanism to control and censure particular behaviors in our society? Do same-sex behaviors occur throughout the animal kingdom, and how does that affect our views about these behaviors?

For those of us who base our belief systems on sacred scriptures, in the fourth chapter we consider what the Torah, the New Testament, the Qur'an, and the teachings of Buddha tell us about homosexuality. As we explore these sacred texts, we also ask whose interpretations of these scriptures we are to follow: Was the sin of Sodom and Gomorrah homosexuality or indifference to the poor and rejected? What do other sacred texts say, and what are the possible interpretations of these various scriptural passages? We also discuss what role, if any, religion and church dogma should play in setting public policy.

In the chapter on ex-gay ministries, we continue our discussion about faith and sexual orientation by looking at how men and women who are conflicted by faith and sexual orientation live their lives and how they try to resolve the conflicts. Can these men and women convert to heterosexuality with the help of prayer and therapy? Are these reparative therapy programs as successful as some would claim or as dangerous as others have told us? How do gay men, lesbians, and bisexuals respond to calls to faith?

The focus of chapter 6 is the lessons we can discover in history in our quest to learn about same-sex behaviors in humans. In particular, we ask whether it's true that homosexuality is linked to the downfall of society, or has homosexuality been an accepted and honored human trait in some of the most successful civilizations within recorded history? How is homosexuality viewed in repressive societies? Why have we written different histories about the same events?

In chapter 7, we look at a question that's often asked when straights encounter effeminate gay men or butch lesbians: why do gay men and lesbians have to be so different? We also explore the accusations that raise fear about what homosexuality might mean for society: Do gay men, lesbians, and bisexuals have higher incidence rates of mental and behavioral disorders and thus threaten society? Are gay men more promiscuous, and is there a higher rate of child molestation (pedophilia and hebophilia) among gay men? We also ask the corollary questions, such as the following: Doesn't society's rejection of LGB individuals have the potential to cause greater emotional and behavioral problems for gay, bisexual and lesbian youth?

What do we know about societies and individuals who hold negative views of homosexuality?

Chapter 8 begins our look at what is called the secret homosexual agenda. Do lesbians and gay men have a secret agenda, or is it an open, well-advertised civil rights movement? Are lesbians and gay men asking for special rights and special protection, or are they seeking our guaranteed rights to life, liberty, and the pursuit of happiness?

In the ninth chapter we consider one of the more controversial elements in the movement for equality—Does *Heather Has Two Mommies* belong on elementary school bookshelves? Should our schools have explicit policies protecting LGB students from harassment? Should we recognize and talk about homosexuality in the curriculum, or do we remain silent on the topic? If we mention homosexuality in the curriculum or allow gay student groups in the school, aren't we supporting and promoting immorality? Do professional ethical standards demand that schools offer policies that protect LGBT students? Is it censorship by omission when textbooks are silent on issues of homosexuality?

In the final chapter, we look back at the answers detailed in the chapters 2–9, calling attention to some recurring themes. Why has this become such a hot-button topic in today's culture, and where will our changes in public attitudes and policy takes us in the future? Is it possible an out-of-the-closet lesbian or gay man could run for president some day?

THE QUEER FOLK WHO ARE COVERED AND THE CONVENTIONS USED

Although the use of the term *queer* in the title is in part a reference to queer theory—a theory that reclaims the word often used to denigrate homosexuals and other sexual and gender minorities (e.g., bisexuals, transsexuals, intersex individuals)—regrettably, this book gives only passing attention to transsexual and intersex persons. These individuals certainly deserve to have their stories told and their issues discussed, but I confess that I lack sufficient background to do so with any degree of depth. Hopefully, those writers who have spent the necessary time and done the research will be able to give voice to these often ignored and harshly treated members of our human family. Because the text doesn't cover transsexuals, the often-used abbreviation LGBT (lesbian, gay, bisexual, and transsexual) has been modified to LGB for the purposes of this narrative, except on those occasions when we are looking at a characteristic that includes transsexual individuals.

As the reader, you will notice a recurring convention throughout these pages: a set of textboxes inserted at various points in each of the chapters. These textboxes provide you with abbreviated stories, summaries of research, and opinions from some of the people I have come across in writing the text—both scholars and friends. These boxes help explicate the topic under discussion, but you could easily bypass them if you so choose. At times, you will also come across references to earlier or upcoming chapters indicating that a specific topic is also discussed, possibly in greater detail, in another part of the text.

SELF-DISCLOSURE, SELF-REFLECTION

As illustrated by the narrative on the tomb of Niankhkhnum and Khnumhotep found in chapter 5 of this text, the stories that we are told are often as dependent on the bias and intentions of the storytellers as the facts on which the stories are based. And as we see in the different interpretations of the passages of Sodom and Gomorrah discussed in chapter 4, the individual messages we find in these stories are strongly influenced by predispositions that we, the readers or listeners, bring with us. With this in mind, I think I owe you the reader a few paragraphs of self-disclosure. I suspect you may also owe yourself a minute or two of reflection on what you bring to our interchange.

A gay male born to caring and devoted parents who were conservative Christians, I learned many of the life lessons that I carry with me today from Dad and Mom. Two of the lessons I learned from my father were the importance of doing the research and the need to challenge myself and my beliefs: in other words, don't be so sure you know what you think you know, and never stop searching for the facts. Considering the rather raucous discussions my father, my older brother, and I would have around the dining room table when Stan Jr. and I were both home from college, I am not sure my mother really appreciated that Dad had taught us this lesson. But this willingness to challenge the norms and the quest for the facts were balanced by a commitment to a life of faith, a lesson we learned from both parents.

With conservative Christianity as a basis for my faith and the need to examine the differing perspectives that were offered to me, I was pretty well destined to cross almost all of the points on the continuum of beliefs about homosexuality, including a year of celibacy and a summer in a committed relationship with a wonderful woman. And my progression across this continuum wasn't neat or orderly, nor was it always appreciated by members of my family. The path I followed was at times influenced by pure emotion and at others by a discipline of thought encouraged by my father and some incredibly talented mentors. I also confess that my first studies on homosexuality were focused on proving the "other" (straight men and women) wrong. More recently, however, this search has been about the joy of discovery, wherever that takes me.

In this personal quest for the candid answers about sexual orientation, I certainly have had to change directions, at times screaming and kicking, when presented with better data. From time to time, these new insights forced me to go back to friends sheepishly asking them to disregard various proclamations on a specific topic surrounding this issue (e.g., origins of sexual orientation, the nature of bisexuality, etc). And although I regret that on occasion I would start down what I now assume to be some wrong paths, I take comfort in knowing that I didn't come to my views easily, and I worked hard to follow the lessons learned, even when it meant reversing course. As could be expected, the lessons learned didn't offer neat, clear-cut answers.

In the end, although this text has certainly been influenced by my personal experiences, it has been important to me to follow the research and scholarship and to give voice to multiple perspectives, accepting incomplete answers even when my natural inclination would have been to wrap things up in a nice neat package. That being said, there is no doubt this is a book written from the perspective of gay male who is a committed believer and who has spent all of his adult life in academia—a gay male who feels a sense of urgency in moving the gay, lesbian, bisexual, and transgendered rights agenda forward, but with honesty and integrity.

A THANK YOU NOTE

Several people were extremely gracious in helping me on my journey as I wrote this book. Working in university and community settings gave me access to five incredibly talented colleagues—Matt Gilg, Lynn Carroll, Carolyn Williams, Janet Owen, and Cindy Watson—who supportively watched over my shoulder as I wrote the biology and genetics, psychology, history, legal, the agenda. and sacred-scriptures segments found throughout the text, offering insights into their respective disciplines. As my genetics coach, Matt deserves special kudos. Melonie Handerson, Shannon McLeish, and Jamie Greenmun were, as always, wonderful proofreaders and editors, and Brandon Eady's patience in formatting parts of the text is greatly appreciated. I gained much from listening to men and women who viewed this topic from very different perspectives—among them were Donald Hayas, Robert Vergenz, Alisia Craddock, and Brice McIntyre. I also want to acknowledge the 13 undergraduate honors students who joined me for a special topics seminar on the material covered in this text. Friends and colleagues, I am in each of your debt.

I also owe a great debt to the scholars who did the research that I am trying to organize and summarize in this text. With a reference list of over 300 works, it would be impossible to mention them all, but I must give thanks to John Boswell for starting me on my journey. When I picked up *Christianity, Social Tolerance, and Homosexuality,* I was looking for a quick answer to a challenge posed by my mother's minister, and what I found was an unquenchable need to study the topic of homosexuality using all of the remarkable tools and resources at my disposal. I wish I had had an opportunity to meet the man before his death.

NOTE

1. The definitions of *queer* are taken from *Dictionary.com Unabridged (v 1.1)*. Retrieved from the Dictionary.com Web site: http://dictionary.reference.com/browse/queer.

2

Who's Queer and Who's Not

Our explorations into the cultural and scientific debates about sexual orientation begin with the most central of questions: What does it mean to be homosexual, bisexual, or heterosexual? On the surface, at least, these questions seem easy enough to answer. After all, the definitions of these words are reasonably well accepted: homosexual—a person who is physically/sexually and emotionally/romantically attracted to members of the same biological sex (Chuck wants to date Tim, and Sue wants to have a family with Carol); heterosexual—a person who is physically and emotionally attracted to members of the opposite biological sex (Erin wants to date Aaron, and Christopher is buying the diamond for Christine); bisexual—a person who is physically and emotionally attracted to both males and females (a few months before Queen started dating Bob she had been in a long-term relationship with Cheryl; Ted is dating both Barry and Barbara). Yet despite this seeming clarity, using these definitions correctly is not always as easy as it might appear. For some of us, the difficulty in applying these terms results from our confusing sexual orientation (whom do I want to sleep with? boys, girls, or both?) with gender identity (do my genitals and my brain agree that I was meant to be a male, or does one say male and the other say female?), or from confusing sexual orientation with gender expression (what clothes do I prefer to wear in public or in private—women's lacy underwear or men's boxers?).

Fortunately, thanks to the efforts of such mainstream personalities as Oprah and Barbara Walters, there is a growing understanding of the differences between, and independence of, sexual orientation and gender identity.

But the work is not finished. Those of us who still confuse these constructs believe that large numbers of, if not all, lesbians see themselves as males and want all of the biology that goes along with *manhood.* Or we mistakenly believe that all men who seek a sex change start out gay and go through the hormone treatments and operations so that they can live as a heterosexual woman, making love to straight men. Neither of these is true. Most homosexual women have no desire to give up their breasts and add a penis, just like most male homosexuals are rather fond of the genitals they have had since birth and don't want them removed. If anything, these men are more apt to want them enlarged.

Although most men who surgically transition into women seek male companionship before and after the treatments, this isn't always the case. Sarah, a friend of mine, began life as Robert, a male who was sexually attracted to women. But despite his attraction to women, Robert felt that there was a woman living inside his brain. Robert became Sarah, and she continued to seek romantic and sexual relationships with women. It was never her intention to sleep with men; she just wanted to be a woman herself. Sarah admits that it was easier to meet women as a male than as a female, but she doesn't regret her choice. Today, her body and her brain feel like they belong together. And they both want to be with another woman, not a man.

Most transsexuals begin living as homosexuals, transitioning to a form of heterosexuality—men who date men seeking to become women who date men, or women who date women transitioning to men who date women. But there are instances of heterosexuals transitioning to homosexuality—men who date women becoming women who date women.

When we confuse sexual orientation with gender expression, we make a different mistake, most often assuming that any male who likes to wear women's clothes must be homosexual. Those of us who make this error are likely to find it very disconcerting when we hear John and his loving wife Susan on the afternoon talk show telling us how John enjoys wearing high heels but still maintains a successful and sexually satisfying marriage with Susan. Of course, Susan admits that she went through some trauma and had many doubts when she found John trying on some of her clothes. But now she accepts this as her husband's quirk, the same as some other heterosexually married women accept the fact that their devoted husbands glance at every pretty skirt that walks by at the shopping mall—off-putting for sure but not necessarily fatal to an otherwise good marriage.

How we want to present ourselves in our public or private lives doesn't necessarily have anything to do with our sexual orientation or our sexual identity. John knows and feels comfortable with being male; he just likes women's clothes. There are drag queens—gay men who dress as women—who feel very comfortable with their male pieces and parts but enjoy dressing as women and performing for others. And yes, there are drag queens who are saving enough money to have their sex change operations. Nature seems to provide any and all possible combinations. There are also lesbians and occasional straight women who feel most comfortable wearing a slightly modified tuxedo to a formal fundraiser, and there are lesbians as well as straight women who enjoy lipstick and long dresses. It certainly seems more likely for a homosexual man to wear women's clothes than a heterosexual man. But nonetheless, we come across both patterns often enough to stop us from jumping to judgment on sexual orientation. With women's clothing styles as varied as they are, in many cases it becomes more difficult to figure out whether a woman is wearing a man's clothes or expressing her individual sense of style.

Although it is regrettable that there isn't nearly as much work done on gender identity and gender expression, reading the work that is available can be terribly fascinating. I recommend *Stone Butch Blues* by Leslie Feinberg as a starting place for the interested reader. I also recommend the novel *Middlesex* by Jeffery Eugenides for those who are interested in getting a glimpse into the lives of people who are born intersex (hermaphrodites)—having ambiguous genitalia and/or showing characteristics of both genders.

Considering all of the possible combinations that can result from the differences in sexual orientation, gender identity, and gender expression, there is no doubt that humans are a very colorful species. Regrettably, when we look at the reactions that society has toward many of these combinations, it reinforces the fact that humans, like most other animals, are a species that feels uncomfortable with and afraid of differences in others.

For those of us who fall into the mainstream—for example, a woman who likes to dress like a woman and to date men—these various combinations can at first be very confusing, frightening, and even off-putting. But the reality is a number of the possible combinations may be equally confusing for the average gay male who likes being a man and likes being with a man. Years ago, as a graduate student, I encountered another transsexual woman who dated other women. I was confused and questioned the logic, if not sanity, of this young coed. It seemed very strange to me. Sadly and humbly, I confess that I even made jokes about the situation. But now, with my having spent time with Sarah, a successful attorney, it seems perfectly clear why both of these individuals, Sarah and my fellow student, took the actions they did. But it did take some effort on my part to get to this point.

DEGREES OF HOMOSEXUALITY

Even after we sort through all of the seemingly endless combinations of orientation, identity, and expression, we continue to confront a number of other problems in operationalizing our definitions of sexual orientation: How do we judge or assess physical and emotional attraction? Is sexual orientation to be determined based on the individual's behavior (sexual acts), her desire (fantasies, dreams), or her self-identity ("I am bi/straight/lesbian")? If and when we come to agreement on the criterion or criteria we use, we also have to decide how strong the attraction needs to be to qualify an individual for one of these categories: If your college roommate Kisha is involved in one sexual act with another woman, does she move from heterosexual to bisexual or homosexual? Or is one opposite-sex fantasy enough to move Cousin Jeff from homosexual to bisexual?

In applying our chosen criteria, we also need to consider the validity of the data we are using in making our decision. After all, can we assume that Phillip, a devout Catholic who is married to a woman, will be honest in telling us about all of his sexual exploits, especially if his behavior, attractions, or self-identity do not comport with church doctrine or societal norms? Is Joanna, the high school student called to the school office, likely to admit that she is sexually and romantically attracted to Kim, one of the girls on her soccer team, when asked by her school counselor? Will the man or woman struggling with his or her sexual orientation answer the anonymous, random telephone survey truthfully? And if we were going to tell an untruth, which way would it go: the heterosexual claiming to be gay or the gay claiming to be heterosexual?

In addition, we need to consider how we recognize or categorize people when they report changes in identity and behavior over time. If Jonah asserts that he is heterosexual early in high school, then claims to be bisexual in college, and finally declares himself homosexual as he's graduating, can we assume he was homosexual throughout but had difficulty admitting it to himself? If Susan was successfully married to a man for 20 years but begins an exclusive relationship with a woman after her husband dies, do we mark her as formerly heterosexual but now homosexual, or do we say she was bisexual the whole time but didn't understand her attractions?

In ancient and classical Greece, it was relatively common for men to have sexual encounters with younger males as well as with their wives, who were also typically younger. There were also men who were noted for having sex only with other men. Despite discussions about these patterns of behavior in their literature, the Greeks had no terms equivalent to *homosexual, bisexual,* or *heterosexual.* Some contemporary scholars have asserted that this lack of vocabulary means that sexual orientation wasn't even considered in Greece and is thus a construct that should not be applied to these societies.

According to Halperin (1989) and other social constructionists and queer theorists, sexual orientation is nothing more than a classification system devised by contemporary societies to rationalize their views of the acceptable and the unacceptable, to differentiate the good from the bad? These theorists assert that the lack of distinction between heterosexual and homosexual within Greek, Roman and other cultures renders these distinctions meaningless in the contexts of these societies.

Scholars who take issue with this theory suggest that Halperin and others gloss over or outright ignore the many classical writings that discuss why some men prefer only male partners whereas others prefer female partners: for example, Martial, Petronius, and Juvenal. These scholars also suggest that queer theorists also ignore the Greek fable on the origins of sexual orientation: At the beginning, there were three types of super-beings. Each of these was made of two parts. Some were made of two sets of male parts, others consisted of two sets of female genitalia, and still others were composed of male and female genitalia. These beings were split in half when they became human. Ever since, these half-completed beings have sought to reconnect with their original other half: men seeking women, women seeking women, and men seeking men (Boswell 1989; Holland 2004; Hubbard 2003).

Another set of concerns, concerns that are more often a topic of conversation for the academics I hang out with at the university than the people in the grocery store where I shop, asks whether questions of sexual orientation are even relevant when studying different cultures. Do those people who engage in same-sex behaviors in one culture fit our contemporary Western definition of homosexual, and should we even attempt to apply contemporary Western words and definitions to other cultures?

Several queer theorists point to the fact that although same-sex behavior is discussed throughout ancient and classic Greek literature as well as depicted in the visual and performing art from these periods, these cultures had no known word for homosexual. Based on such findings, these same scholars suggest that if the Greeks found no need to classify people based on the gender of their sexual partners, why would we impose our classifications systems on them?

In a similar fashion, other writers note that in the Sambian culture of Papua New Guinea, young boys and male adolescents were expected to have sex with each other until they reached adulthood, when they would enter into heterosexual marriages.[1] Are we to consider these boys homosexual? Or is the term meaningless in the Sambian culture? For most of us, these questions may seem very removed from our day-to-day life and all too much like some of those questions our professors asked when we were in Philosophy or Sociology 101.

John and Janice Baldwin (1989) and Gilbert Herdt and Robert Stoller (1989) report on a well-accepted practice found among the Sambinas of Papua New Guinea. In this culture, young boys were separated from their families sometime between 7 and 10 years of age, most often unwillingly. Living in male-only clubhouses, the young boys were required to perform fellatio on male adolescents who lived with them. Swallowing the sperm is assumed to bring the prepubescent boys into manhood. The adolescents, having begun to come into manhood, must share their semen with their younger club mates. When mature enough, these adolescents leave the clubhouse for heterosexual marriage.

In describing this phenomenon, both sets of authors comment on the fact that some men continue to engage in same-sex activities after leaving the clubhouse and throughout their adulthood. The authors refer to these adults as participating in aberrant behavior and seemingly dismiss the idea of adult homosexuality in the culture.

WHAT DO WE USE TO IDENTIFY SEXUAL ORIENTATION: BEHAVIOR, DESIRE, OR IDENTITY?

When our true behavior, desire, and self-identity are all congruent, conclusions about our sexual orientation seem evident. Your coworker Saul has sex with and fantasizes exclusively about men, and he labels himself as gay. He has been living this way for the past 10 years. It's probably safe for you to mark Saul's name down in the homosexual column. Similarly, Sarah, Saul's sister-in-law, has sex with and fantasizes about men, labeling herself as straight. She has been married to Saul's brother for 15 years. Sarah is probably best thought of as heterosexual. Despite the fact that such alignment (behavior, desire, and identity) occurs for most people, this is by no means always the case.

There are a number of humans who exhibit some dissonance among these characteristics. For some of us, behavior can be separated from identity or attraction. Our attractions and specific behaviors may indicate one category of sexual orientation, but we may, for a number of different reasons, loudly profess a different identity. In some cases, especially among adolescents and young adults, alignment among these variables may come about as a result of maturation or as the individual "comes out of the closet," but this certainly is not an absolute given.[2]

In a national study of sexual attitudes and behaviors, Edward Laumann and his fellow researchers found that 145 (10%) of 1,410 American adult males surveyed reported that they (a) had engaged in sexual activity with other men, (b) felt desire for or sexual attraction to men, and/or (c) identified themselves as homosexual or bisexual. Only 35 of these 145 men said that they fit all three of these criteria: behavior, desire, and identity. In contrast, 32 of these men indicated that even though they had engaged in male-on-male sexual activity in adulthood, they had no sexual attraction to men. Sixty-three of these men indicated that although they had same-sex desires, they had not engaged in same-sex behaviors and did not identify as homosexual or bisexual. And 3 of these men reported thinking of themselves as bisexual or homosexual, but had never engaged in sex with another male.[3]

Among the 1,749 women who completed this survey, 150 (8.6%) acknowledged having had sex with another adult woman, being attracted to other women, and/or identifying as homosexual or bisexual. Only 23 of these 150 women reported meeting all three of these criteria. Eighty-eight of these women reported being attracted to other women, but at the same time they told the interviewer that they had never engaged in same-sex activities as an adult nor did they think of themselves as bisexual or homosexual.

Lisa Diamond (2003), a researcher working with non-heterosexual women, and Ritch Savin-Williams (2005), who writes about adolescents and young adults, point to a question that is not uncommon among different minorities: "What do we call ourselves?"

There is a small but vocal group of individuals who engage in same-sex behaviors and find themselves attracted to same-sex partners that question and reject the terms gay, lesbian, homosexual and bisexual. Some are opting for terms such as unlabeled, pansexual, queerboi, bi-lesbian, polysexual, and so on. Adopting different labels or descriptors serves various purposes for different groups. For some it is a rejection of terms that the individual feels have been pressed on them by a repressive society. Others believe that none of the existing terms quite capture who they are.

In his book *Androphilia: A Manifesto,* Jack Malebranche suggests that the term *gay* denotes cultural practices that have nothing to do with same-sex love between two men and suggests that the term *androphilia* should be used to differentiate same-sex love between men from gay culture. He doesn't deny an attraction to men or the term *homosexuality,* but he does resent being put into a group that follows some of the cultural practices he associates with the word *gay.*

When we look at other subcultures, we can find similar shifts in vocabulary. The term *colored* was understood as a racist term, and *negro* became the term of choice. In turn, *negro* gave way to *black.* Then we saw the introduction of the terms Afro-American and African American as well as the continued use of black. We began with *handicapped* and moved to *disabled.* And we see terms such as *visually challenged* and *developmentally delayed.*

Based on Laumann and his colleagues' data, it is apparent that a percentage of us might be considered heterosexual, bisexual, or homosexual using one measure but would not be considered so if we applied one or both of the other two criteria. As a result, we are left with the question of which criterion to use for classifying someone as homosexual, bisexual, or heterosexual. Ought it be the public or private label we place on ourselves, or should it be the thoughts that run through our minds, or do we use the sex acts in which we engage?

Identity

Some writers suggest that it is appropriate to use self-identification as the critical criterion: "you are what you think you are or what you claim to be." Lisa Diamond makes a strong case for using this standard when she writes about the shifting identity among women. In her 10-year longitudinal study, Diamond found that although many non-heterosexual women maintained a stable sexual orientation, a significant number of these women experienced fluidity or fluctuations in their identity. These changes occurred over time and followed multiple trajectories: lesbian to bisexual, lesbian to heterosexual, and so on.[4]

Yet despite the evidence presented in Diamond's research and the call by some to use self-identification as the primary indicator of sexual orientation, it is doubtful that even the most politically correct of us would utilize this criterion as the gold standard in every case. When Senator "I-have-been-married-and-faithful-to-my-wife-of-18-years" is caught in bed with another man, can he say, "I am not homosexual!" and expect us to believe him? This question is especially poignant when records indicate prior occurrences of such behavior. In a situation such as this, the person's denials seem self-serving and hollow and quite frankly insulting to those of us who are homosexual and see no reason to deny this characteristic of our being. And what of the married man who is living on the down-low, regularly having sex with other men—do we accept his denial of homosexuality or bisexuality as proof of his heterosexuality? In both of these cases, denials of being gay, if *gay* means belonging to a cultural group within society, may be plausible. But disclaimers about being homosexual or bisexual when these are judged by behavior and attraction seem to test the individual's credibility and integrity.

Behavior

Although many of us might be inclined to use documented behavior in making judgments about the senator or the man living on the down-low, we recognize that there are other situations in which sexual acts fail as an indicator of sexual orientation. In such instances, self-identity or attraction might provide better criteria.

When San Quentin prisoners engage in same-sex activities, we willingly accept that these behaviors may be situational aberrations that have no bearing on the individuals' sexual orientation. For Scar-Faced Sam, the 45-year-old, 210-pound, assertive, repeat convict, his male-on-male sexual encounters in prison might be classified as acts of rape or as impersonal sex meant to establish dominance or satisfy unfulfilled sexual urges, but not as a measure of his sexual orientation. For Pretty-Boy Harry, the 20-year-old heterosexual male who is forced to assume the passive-receptive role, these acts may also fail to provide any information about sexual orientation. Under such circumstances, self-identity tells us more about orientation than the behavior.

In a similar vein, using the definitions in the beginning of this chapter, the 25 percent of American boys who engage in same-sex activities with one or more male peers[5] or the young Arandan boys who have sex with their uncles as their introduction into manhood[6] should not be considered homosexual or bisexual. These are acts of exploration or exploitation, not acts that define orientation.

So if the presence of a behavior is an insufficient marker under certain circumstances (e.g., Scar-Faced Sam) but the lead indicator of sexual orientation on other occasions (e.g., Senator "I-have-been married-and-faithful-to-my-wife-of-18-years"), is the absence of behavior conclusive evidence for eliminating a category of sexual orientation? Is Father Michael, who remains celibate, to be thought of as asexual—a person without sexual interest? In cases where behavior is suppressed out of a sense of a higher good, sexual orientation, be it heterosexuality, homosexuality, or bisexuality, still exists and may still help define a person and her or his outlooks.

Desire

If neither self-identity nor behavior provides us with the definitive marker for sexual orientation, should we use attraction or desire as the gold standard? If reported honestly and accurately, it might seem so. However, even here we have to be careful. There are women who identify themselves as straight, contently living what would be considered heterosexual lives, but who from time to time fantasize about other women when they are enjoying sex with their husbands.[7] These women have no desire to fulfill their fantasies. Similarly, there are gay men who will on occasion fantasize about heterosexual coupling during sex with a male partner but who have no interest in acting on the fantasy. Should either of these groups be considered bisexual? Probably not, if we are talking only about a fantasy life with no desire to act it out.

STRAIGHT TALK

So where are we in understanding the answer to our original question: what does it mean to be heterosexual, bisexual, or homosexual? In some ways it may feel like we are traveling through one of those mazes that appear in paper-and-pencil puzzle books, the ones where with each turn you find yourself at another road block. But how do we get out of the maze? Where is the exit that leads us to the answer?

To begin our exit from the maze, it's important to remember the turns that lead us to the dead ends most quickly. First, although often ignored in the literature, having sex with a same-sex partner does not necessarily meet our definition of homosexual or bisexual: "attraction to." All that it means is that a person had one or more same-sex experiences. "Pretty-Boy Harry" and the boys from Sambia weren't homosexuals who converted to heterosexuality. Many of Pretty-Boy Harry's friends in prison and most of the Sambian youth started out heterosexual and remained heterosexual throughout the period of their same-sex experiences. Some started out homosexual and remained homosexual after they left prison or the boy's clubhouse. Likewise, if you experimented with your same-sex preadolescent cousin or neighbor, that doesn't mean that you were necessarily homosexual or bisexual. All it means is that you, along with 25 percent or so of your friends, broke a societal taboo. You played sex games with a same-sex peer, but hopefully you made sure your parents didn't walk in on you.

In most cases, being homosexual also doesn't mean that you want to change your biological sex. Most homosexuals revel in their gender, taking pride in their genitals and in those of their same-sex partners. Of course, there are some gay men and lesbians who have opposite gender identities. And that plays no part in the definitions of homosexuality or bisexuality.

Now that we have some sense of the dead ends in our maze, let me suggest that in finding our exit, we choose a path in which homosexuality, bisexuality, and heterosexuality don't exist as three absolute and discrete categories. As is true with many human characteristics, sexual orientation would seem to be a complex continuum. Alfred Kinsey's work suggests that there are virtually an infinite number of gradations between being exclusively heterosexual and exclusively homosexual.[8] This is not all that dissimilar from human traits such as height, hair color, and intellect, to name a few. When does the natural blonde become a strawberry blonde, and when does he become a redhead? And is our assessment of his hair color best made after he has been inside in the winter or when he has spent the summer in the sun? In a similar vein, when do we consider Cassandra a heterosexual as opposed to a bisexual, and what actions or criteria move her to being a homosexual?

In acknowledging the complexity of this particular trait, Diamond and others have suggested that we consider using three different assessments and three different classifications for each individual: sexual orientation based on behavior, sexual orientation based on romantic attraction, and sexual orientation based on self-identification.[9] Although 91 to 92 percent of us would fall at very similar points on all three of these continuums, 8 to 9 percent of us would show a reasonably significant level of incongruence on where we place ourselves on these scales. Jared could be exclusively homosexual in

In introducing his Heterosexual Homosexual Rating Scale, Alfred Kinsey suggested six different ratings on his continuum of sexual orientation:

0. = exclusively heterosexual

1. = predominately heterosexual and only incidentally homosexual

2. = predominately heterosexual but more than incidentally homosexual

3. = equally heterosexual and homosexual

4. = predominately homosexual but more than incidentally heterosexual

5. = predominately homosexual and only incidentally heterosexual

6. = exclusively homosexual

Individuals who have a rating of 0 or 1 would be considered heterosexual, ratings of 5 or 6 would equate to homosexual, and ratings 2, 3, and 4 would be labeled as bisexual (Kinsey, Pomeroy, and Martin 1948, 638).

Of course, we could have an ongoing debate on what *predominantly*, *exclusively*, and *incidentally* mean.

attraction and bisexual in behavior and label himself as heterosexual; Julie could be bisexual in attractions but exclusively heterosexual in behavior and identify herself as heterosexual.

In contrast to the multidimensional approach, Kinsey suggested that we analyze the behavioral and psychological (affectional) attractions for each person and come to a decision on a single rating.[10] Such a unidimensional classification system certainly does make it easier for discussions with the people we might meet at my grocery store: "Yes, my son Robert is living with a man, but he considers himself bisexual as opposed to homosexual because he occasionally has heterosexual fantasies" versus "My son Robert is gay and happily living with a wonderful partner." Yet the multidimensional approach does reflect the complexity of human behaviors, emotions, and self-perceptions.

Both approaches have merit and may provide alternative exits out of our maze. When there is major congruence between affection and behavior, the best exit is easy—we go with one term: homosexual, heterosexual, or bisexual. When there is dissonance between the terms, and we aren't involved in scientific study, in our day-to-day life most of us would still be best served by one term, using the overriding characteristic to define the individual, à la Kinsey. If, however, we are acting as scholars using the data for scientific study, there is great value in using a multidimensional approach, measuring each of the characteristics separately, if for no other reason than you are likely to get more honest answers than when you try to force respondents into a single choice.

If you are making a single choice, attraction and behavior will more often than not trump self-identity because identity often trails behind the other two characteristics. When there is a conflict between attraction and behavior, a closer look at each is needed. If Leslie is pulled to act on homosexual attractions but fears the consequences, she could well be labeled homosexual or bisexual. We need to know about what else turns Leslie on. But Peter, who is "just experimenting" or looking for a quick sexual outlet at a gay bathhouse each and every time he goes out of town, is probably not heterosexual, even though he will protest that he never kisses the men with whom he has sex.

When we choose the multidimensional approach as our exit point, past studies leave no doubt that the greatest number of humans will be on the heterosexual side on all three continuums. But those humans who fall somewhere between bisexual and homosexual on only one of the three scales are more likely to do so based on desire or behavior than on self-identity. Not surprisingly, humans seem to accept the label only after they have acknowledged the feelings and taken a dip in the pool, as it were.

As with so many of those paper and pencil mazes, our exit point could have served as our entry point: being homosexual denotes that you have a strong and almost exclusive sexual and psychological attraction to people of your same gender. You may or may not act on this attraction, and at times, you may deny it to yourself—if, for example, your culture doesn't provide you with the language to label yourself, your homosexual self-identity conflicts with your self-identity as a good Muslim, or you fear the societal repercussions of being known as gay or lesbian—but the attraction is still there. Being heterosexual means you have strong and almost exclusive sexual and psychological attraction to individuals of the opposite gender. You too may or may not act on these attractions, but they are there. However, it's highly unlikely in such heterosexual cases that you will hide from the label. After all, it makes you a part of the bigger and most socially acceptable club. And to be bisexual means you have the best and worst of both worlds—your attractions may move from one gender to the other even if your behaviors don't.

These attractions may occur in the same time frame, or they may change over time. But in donning the label *bisexual,* you are also likely to be labeled by others as being unsure or being in transition to a self-awareness of your homosexuality. And for some self-professed bisexuals, the "in transition" label may be true. But for others there is no uncertainty or transition; there is lifelong bisexuality.

Whichever of these categories humans perceive they belong in, it is possible that they may shift positions on that scale at some later point in life. Adjustments to our recognized attractions, behaviors, and self-identity could be the result of greater self-knowledge, or they might signal a shift in our inner being. Research provides us with countless self-accounts that demonstrate the first pattern—commonly referred to as the process of coming out. In coming out we recognize bisexual or homosexual traits over a span of time, becoming more comfortable and more vocal about them. For some men and women this process may occur quickly in adolescence; for others it can take decades.

At the same time, researchers such as Lisa Diamond and Ritch Savin-Williams are uncovering a growing body of evidence that suggests the second pattern (shift in desire) occurs in some cases. As opposed to a discovery of the inner being, for a minority of homosexuals and bisexuals, there may be an actual shift in the inner being. This seems to be true for women more so than for men.

HOW MANY HOMOSEXUALS CAN
FIT INTO A POLLING BOOTH?

Our attempts to identify the percentage of bisexuals and homosexuals in any given population have proven to be frustrating and contentious to say the least. It's almost as if those of us on both sides of the debates on sexual orientation want the number to remain unknown to serve our own political interests. Our arguments often result from opposing ideas about the genesis of homosexuality and from questions about the power that homosexuals and bisexuals may wield in the polling booth and the marketplace.

Those of us who hold differing points of view on the origins of homosexuality mistakenly believe that we have a vested interest in stacking the deck when it comes to the incidence rates of homosexuality. Many of us who claim homosexuality is a natural phenomenon believe that our argument is stronger if 10 percent of the population is homosexual rather than 1 percent. In contrast, those who feel that homosexuality is an aberration of nature or an environmentally induced syndrome would prefer to see the number at 1 percent or below.

The point we are missing is that the rate of occurrence tells us nothing about the origin. Rates of environmentally caused cancers are considerably higher than the 1 percent incidence rate of red hair, a genetically determined characteristic.[11] Of course, if you lived in Scotland or Ireland, you might find it difficult to believe that only 1 percent of humans have red hair. But then again, if you lived in the Castro area of San Francisco, a gay mecca, you might think that at least 90 percent of the world population was gay or lesbian.

The reality is that if the incidence rates of homosexuality were .001 percent, it still could be a natural occurring event as opposed to an aberration of nature or environmentally induced. And if it was as high as 100 percent, it could still have an environmental origin. Incidence doesn't document origin.

George W. Bush won the 2000 Presidential election by 537 votes. Exit polls indicate that 57,000 or 25% of Florida's gay and lesbian voters pushed the lever for George Bush. Had these Log Cabin Republicans (the name of the gay and lesbian Republicans) gone the other way, Al Gore would have been elected president (Phelps n.d.).

Considering what happened to the gay rights agenda during George W.'s term in office, it seems ironic that Bush's victory could have been taken away from him had Al Gore captured 100 percent of the homosexual vote in Florida instead of the estimated 90 percent that he did get.

If I were a Log Cabin Republican who voted for Bush, during his tenure in office I don't think I would have publicly admitted it at many dinner parties with gay or lesbian friends, especially if my name were Chad. In such a case the term "hanging chad" could have taken on a whole new meaning.

However, it is not difficult to understand the arguments about the size of the LGB population when we think of economic and political power. Increased prevalence equates to increased power, especially when we consider the voting booth and the shopping mall. If 10 percent of the population is homosexual or bisexual, then they become a much more potent voting block — one that many of our politicians can't afford to ignore. Likewise, if 10 percent of the population were homosexual and bisexual, we would become an extremely compelling economic force for industry and for marketers. These facts notwithstanding, it is important to remember that many elections are lost by 1 to 2 percent of the vote. But it's also important to note that the voting power of gays and lesbians has not stopped state constitutional bans on same-sex marriage. Having 5 percent of the overall U.S. population isn't sufficient to guarantee a political victory in a given area. It still takes alliances with larger groups of the population to bring that about.

Advertisers are also catching on to the fact that whether by pure numbers or because of dollars in disposable income, homosexuals and bisexuals have a great deal of purchasing power. Several years ago, evangelical Christians threatened to boycott Disney theme parks because the parks had collaborated with gay and lesbian groups to set aside a weekend for Gay Days at Disney. When Mickey's corporate executives did the math, they realized they had more to gain from welcoming gays and lesbians to the parks than they had to lose from what would be an ineffectual boycott. Their calculations proved to be right. In fact, they were so correct that a number of other family-centered amusement parks followed suit, and for one weekend every year in June, Orlando's amusement parks become a virtual sea of same-sex couples and single lesbians and gay men. It didn't matter whether 1 percent or 10 percent of the population was lesbian and gay; they held enough purchasing power to get Disney's attention.

In 2007 the city of Philadelphia filmed and aired a travel advertisement that first showed a set of would-be historic love letters between two people, presumably written in the 1700s.

At the end of the commercial, the viewer finally got to see the two lovers meet in Philadelphia circa 1776. They were two very handsome young men in colonial dress. After all, it is the city of brotherly love.

If you look at mainstream gay publications (*mainstream gay* may seem like an oxymoron to some readers) or at the programming and advertisements that appear on gay- and lesbian-focused cable television networks, you'll see that the travel industry has certainly caught on to the spending power of this 1 to 10 percent segment of the population. Cities, car rental companies, hotels, and other corporate interests often place ads specifically tailored to the LGB (lesbian, gay, bisexual) population.

Counting the Queers

With the battles over origins as well as political and economic power providing an ongoing hum of background noise, we continue to fall far short of agreement on the incidence rates of homosexuality and bisexuality. To some degree, this lack of consensus rests on the fact that in the United States we have chosen, with political intent, not to use the largest data-gathering tool at our disposal to help answer the question: the U.S. Census. In the 2000 census, the Census Bureau did ask one question on how many same-sex partner households there were in America, a major step in the direction of capturing data related to sexual orientation. But the census failed to ask several other questions that would have given us a much more robust picture of sexual orientation in America, including how many of the same-sex households were gay or lesbian as opposed to say two heterosexual women who might be living together with their children for economic reasons.

Inclusion of other more direct questions was blocked by a number of federal lawmakers, at least two of whom have left the House and the Senate under clouds of suspicion about their own sexual orientation. In contrast, Britain has conducted two nationally financed studies, first in 1990 and again in 2000, providing us with data that offer a very different calculus on sexual orientation from what we had in the past. And countries such as France and Australia have taken similar actions.

Truth in Labeling

Even the best designed population surveys continue to present two problems that we have already discussed. In determining prevalence rates we still have no agreement on what constitutes homosexuality: behavior, attraction, or self-identity. And as documented in the various studies, these different definitions produce significantly different figures on sexual orientation. Recognizing this lack of universal agreement, the best of these studies capture data on at least two of these three dimensions, leaving interpretation up to the reader. The "let's keep the rate low for our political purposes" crowd is then free to use the self-identity number as the one it will quote. And "the bigger the number, the better" gang can use the attraction or behavior numbers, or they can include everyone who appears in any of the three categories combined when they cite the study.

The other factor that confounds our ability to get a clear handle on how many heterosexuals, homosexuals, and bisexuals there are in any given population is that we don't know how accurately respondents report these types of data. There is good reason to suspect that some may intentionally report data inaccurately because of unfounded fear of disclosure, whereas others may unintentionally report incorrect data as a result of self-denial and their internal struggle to understand who they are.

Fortunately, although self-denial and underreporting are still likely to be common practices among homosexuals and bisexuals, comparisons of the data found in the 1990 and 2000 British studies suggest that there may be a shift in attitudes about acknowledging and self-reporting same-sex behaviors and attractions. After all, with so many contemporary television shows including one or more gay or lesbian characters, it is becoming easier to report same-sex encounters, at least on the anonymous survey, if not to your parents or clergy. In 1990, 3.7 percent of British male respondents reported having had sex with other men. When the study was repeated in 2000, 6.3 percent of the male respondents said that they had engaged in sex with a same-gender partner. In 1990, only 1.9 percent of women said that they had had sex with another woman. Ten years later, 5.7 percent of the female respondents reported that they had participated in same-sex behaviors.[12] These incredible changes in the percentage of respondents who reported same-sex behaviors, especially among women, evidence either a new openness in acknowledging same-sex behaviors or an increase in acting on the desires that were hidden. Most likely the upward climb in these numbers reflects a little of both. Yes, the times, they are a changing. But even with these reporting shifts, we can assume that there continues to be an unknown level of underreporting.

Give Me the Facts Ma'am, Only the Facts

So what is the number or percentage of homosexuals within the population? Is it 1 percent or fewer, or is it 10 percent or more?

Alfred Kinsey, a pioneer in research on human sexuality, is credited with the first attempts at assessing the prevalence rates of homosexuality. Often cited as saying that 10 percent of the American male population was homosexual, what Kinsey and his colleagues in fact did report was that 10 percent of the males they studied were *more or less homosexual for at least three years between the ages of 16 and 55,* and 4 percent of white males he studied *were exclusively homosexual throughout their entire lives.*[13] These data are often cited as the basis for the common estimate that 10 percent of the population is homosexual.

Unfortunately, despite some of the strengths of his surveys and interviews, Kinsey's sampling techniques left much to be desired and have justifiably generated a number of criticisms about the accuracy of his numbers. The male participants Kinsey and his colleagues used in their study were predominantly white, they voluntarily signed up to be in a study on sexual attitudes and activities, and they included a higher percentage of college students than would be expected as well as an overrepresentation of volunteers who had been in the prison system.

As any first-year doctoral student in the social sciences could tell you, using Kinsey's sample to make generalizations about the behaviors of American males in general is subject to question. Using his data to make predictions about the rate of homosexuality in America would be similar to us testing a sample of students from private preparatory schools and a set of students in chess clubs at public high schools and using their, and only their, test scores to determine the mathematical ability among U.S. high school students. It would be logically and statistically indefensible to use the achievement scores from these highly select students to draw conclusions about the math skills across all American high school students.

Since Kinsey's initial research of male sexuality and his research on sexuality among American women, several studies have been conducted to confirm, disprove, or provide better data than what Kinsey and his colleagues reported. Although the results of these studies vary, together they begin to provide us with minimum estimates for incidence rates of same-sex behavior and same-sex attraction. They fail, however, to paint bright lines between homosexuality and bisexuality.

In addition, because of participant reluctance to report honestly on these topics, we should limit our use of the percentages provided in these studies to setting the floor for estimated rates of homosexuality, as opposed to defining an absolute percentage. To use the data otherwise would be to engage in an error of probable underestimation, at least equal to or greater than the error of probable overestimation found in Kinsey's original study.

Using five of the best and largest random sample surveys, we are able to calculate estimated minimum percentages for male and female homosexuality/bisexuality, when the criterion is self-identification, expressed desire and attraction, or behavior. These five studies include a 1990s survey of 3,917 men and 4,827 women selected from across the United States. The second study crossed national boundaries and included respondents from the United States (1,288 men and 634 women), Britain (1,137 men and 696 women), and France (1,506 men and 788 women). The third and fourth studies were both carried out in Britain, one in 1990 (8,335 men and 10,412 women) and the other in 2000 (3,392 men and 4,747 women). The fifth and most recent study was conducted in Australia and New Zealand (10,173 men and 9,134 women). A summary of the data from these studies appears in the table at the end of this chapter.

Considering the data from all of these studies, it seems safe to estimate that somewhere between 4 and 6 percent of males are homosexual or bisexual. For women the range would conservatively be between 2 and 5 percent. In light of the probabilities of underreporting, these figures may in fact climb higher. These estimates are not that different from Kinsey's data on lifelong homosexuality but are clearly less than the most often quoted 10 percent figure.

It is interesting to note the data for the 1990 British study compared to the 2000 study. Both of these studies used the same techniques but were conducted 10 years apart. In looking at the results, across the board, we notice an upturn in percentages from one decade to the next for men and women. This might be the result of an actual escalation in same-sex activity (increased social approval leading to a freedom to act on desire), a greater willingness to report the activity (increased social acceptance leading to greater freedom to admit desire and behavior), or an increased self-recognition of what's happening in the individual respondents' lives (increased societal awareness leading to a higher likelihood of self-awareness). Each or some combination of these variables probably contributes to the change in results. With the change in public acceptance and the greater open dialogue in Western societies, it does become easier for a homosexual or bisexual to accept, acknowledge, and act on her or his attractions to same-gender partners. These results may serve as fodder for those of us who oppose equality for lesbians and gay men and thrill those of us who are pro–gay rights advocates: "Isn't it frightening to know that we are creating a culture that encourages immorality?" versus "Isn't in heartening to know that we are moving forward with allowing people to be who they were meant to be?" Some of us see disorder; some of us see discovery.

OTHER THINGS WE LEARNED

The data from these studies provide us with strong evidence supporting a long-held assumption that the rates of homosexuality and bisexuality differ for women and men. In virtually every study, men report greater rates of homosexuality overall than do women, regardless of definition. Previous studies, and most of the studies included in Appendix A, lead us to hypothesize that males among us are more likely to be homosexual than the females among us. Although not apparent from the data presented in the five studies covered here, women are, however, assumed to display higher rates of long-term bisexuality. For many men bisexuality appears to be a stage in the self-acceptance and coming-out processes.

In a recently completed study (Egan, Edelman, and Sherrill 2008, 6) conducted by Hunter College and the Human Rights Campaign, 68.4 percent of nonheterosexual men identified themselves as gay or homosexual and 31.6 percent referred to themselves as bisexual. For women the figures were reversed: 34.7 percent thought of themselves as homosexual, gay, or lesbian and 65.3 percent referred to themselves as bisexual.

The details about the rates of homosexuality and bisexuality in different countries from these and other surveys present us with some interesting, if not all that surprising, facts. Homosexuals, and most especially gay men, are not distributed equally across any given national landscape. These men and women tend to leave small-town America, England, and France and move to the big city (San Francisco, New York, London, Paris) or to select smaller towns (Key West, Provincetown, Brighton Beach, the south part of St. Tropez) that have reputations for being homocentric or gay enclaves. Predictably, gay men and lesbians seek to live in areas where they are well accepted and can thrive both professionally and personally. If you look in these cities and towns, the gay and lesbian populations will, at times, exceed Kinsey's often disputed 10 percent. Laumann and his colleagues found that in the 12 largest U.S. metropolitan areas, homosexual men made up between 9.2 and 16.7 percent of the overall male population.[14] To paraphrase Judy Garland, the gay icon of the 1960s and 1970s who starred in the *Wizard of Oz,* Toto, I've got a feeling we are not in Kansas anymore; I think this is San Francisco. For women the rate of self-identified bisexuality and homosexuality grew slightly higher in major cities.

What may be less readily apparent is that when gay men relocate into a city or a sector within the city, as opposed to mayhem and destruction, these men often bring culture and commerce. The truth is, if you want to find the art scene, good food, and often a great university, find a homosexual and follow him or her. They will lead you to some of the most interesting and cosmopolitan places in the country, including the best dance bars. If, on the other hand, you are happier with paintings of Elvis, the greasy spoon diner and a so-so junior college you might want to pick a town where the policies are hostile to homosexuality. Let me offer a word of caution, if it's late at night and the gay male is wearing heavy black leather drag, you might consider waiting to find another gay male to follow. (Now, before any of you write a scathing letter, I know this is stereotyping, but not necessarily without some basis. See chapter 7, "Pardon Me, But Do You Have Size 13 Toe Shoes in Stock?")

Our surveys also tell us that on average, homosexuals have higher incomes than the population in general and are more likely to hold professional positions. But if you are homosexual, before you celebrate these facts, you need to keep in mind two interesting and disturbing footnotes. First, although the prospects of a higher-than-average income is a reality, as with every population, there are those homosexual individuals who are outliers and don't fit the generalization. In this particular instance, there are large numbers of homosexual and bisexual youth who have been kicked out of the house and are barely scraping by with what they have. Some of these young women and men are living and working on the streets. We cannot assume that homosexuality is a ticket to financial security. And I would suggest that middle- and upper-class homosexuals and their heterosexual allies should make concerted efforts to find ways to help these at-risk-youth.

A second interesting, but not often reported, artifact is that although overall average incomes are higher for homosexual men and women, this is because they tend to be better educated. But when you compare homosexual males to their heterosexual counterparts performing the same job, you are likely to find the homosexual male earning a lower salary than his straight peer. If his heterosexual counterpart is married, the salary difference between the straight guy and the gay guy will average 23 percent. And the gay guy doesn't come out on top. It seems there may be a lavender ceiling.

On the other hand, when you compare the salaries of homosexual and heterosexual women filling the same role, especially if it is a professional position, you will find that the homosexual female often earns a slightly higher salary.[15] In the eyes of their bosses, gay men don't seem to require the same incomes as their married male peers, or maybe they aren't seen as likely to move on to the competitor. After all, shouldn't they feel blessed to work for a company that loves them and offers domestic partner benefits? Lesbians, on the other hand, may be seen as more career-oriented than their heterosexual counterparts. But even here gay rights supporters will want to temper their enthusiasm. Although lesbians make more than straight women, they still earn less than male heterosexual peers. The glass ceiling is still lower than the lavender ceiling.

STRAIGHT TALK

Those of us in the LGB community need to stop quoting or, if you would, misquoting Kinsey when talking about the percent of the population that is bisexual and homosexual. Ten percent makes good headlines, but we don't have and may never have solid evidence to document a statistic like that. Based on today's evidence, we should be comfortable with an estimate that 5 percent of the population fits our definition for bisexuality and homosexuality.

Two questions we might ask ourselves are (1) will this number increase, and (2) will we get better data to separate bisexuality from homosexuality? As society becomes more comfortable with homosexuality and bisexuality, it's highly likely that more LGB people will become comfortable with their own sexual orientation and will become more open about acknowledging it in surveys. We may also choose to use more sophisticated and comprehensive ways of assessing and verifying prevalence in the population. As far as separating people into homosexual versus bisexual, we will always have some difficulty when we get to the edges of either group. I have slept with and even had ongoing and caring relationships with women, but I don't consider myself to be bisexual. We will have the same difficulty in separating certain levels of bisexuality from heterosexuality. As much as part of my personality might love to see definitive numbers, I have come to understand that the actual numbers are really less important than we might think.

Would we as a society predicate granting civil rights based on the percentage of population that fits into a given category? Consider the fact that 0.4 percent of the U.S. population is deaf, 0.2 percent of the world's population is Jewish, and 0.4 percent of the Iranian population is Christian. Do you need to be 10 percent of a population to have your human rights protected, or is it 5 percent? Consider the fact that elections are often won by 1 and 2 percent of the vote. If 537 of the 57,000 gay and lesbian Floridians who voted for George W. Bush had gone to the mall or Home Depot instead of the polling booth on that Tuesday in 2000, America would be a different country today. Five hundred and thirty-seven LGB people changed history by going to the polls and punching out George W.'s chad.

As we think about numbers, we also need to remember that if we live in a community with a great cultural and art scene, we are more likely to have a gay male or lesbian standing in the backyard or sitting on the condo balcony next to ours. And these men and women are demonstrably adding to the economic health of our community.

NOTES

1. Baldwin and Baldwin 1989; Herdt and Stoller 1989.
2. In her theory, Diamond (2003) suggests that we must think of affection separate from sexual desire.
3. Laumann, Gagnon, Michael, and Michaels 1994, 298–301. Similar results for men and women have been found in national studies conducted in Australia and New Zealand (Smith, Rissel, Ritchers, Grulich, and deVisser 2003) and in Britain and France (Sell, Wells, and Wypij 1995; Wellings, Wadsworth, and Johnson 1994).
4. Diamond 2007.
5. In his 2003 article, Goldstein suggests that as many as 25 percent of young males will engage in some sexual activity with a same-gender peer as they discover their own sexual identity. These activities often consist of mutual masturbation. Sixty percent of young males who will grow up to be gay will have engaged in these activities.
6. Ford and Beach 1951.
7. Bickham, O'Keefe, Baker, Berhie, Kommor, and Harper-Dorton 2007; Hamer and Copeland 1998.
8. Kinsey, Pomeroy, and Martin 1948, 638–47.
9. Diamond 2003.
10. Kinsey, Pomeroy, and Martin 1948, 647.
11. Nelson 2004.
12. Wellings et al. 1994; Erens, McManus, Prescott, and Field 2001. These two surveys of sexual attitudes and behavior provide a unique opportunity to examine the shifts in behavior and attitudes over a decade in one country.
13. Kinsey, Pomeroy, and Martin 1948, 651. In this section Kinsey also reports a great deal of information on early same-sex encounters, incidence rates for bachelors, single incidences of same-sex behavior, and so on.
14. Laumann et al. 1994, 306.
15. Elmslie and Telbadi 2007.

3

The Origins of Sexual Orientation

What induces Jane to love John, while Betty can't stop thinking about Barb, and Craig would be happy to be with Christine or Christopher? This is one of those queer questions on which the court of public opinion has flip-flopped back and forth throughout history; with the debates about the origin of sexual orientation extending at least as far back as Plato's Symposium.

The current and most popular theories on genetic and hormonal origins of sexual orientation versus origins in early childhood development and parenting are certainly not new. The genetic and hormonal theories can be traced back to the mid-1800s and early 1900s in the writings of Karl Ulrich and Magnus Hirchfeld. At the same time, the theory that homosexuality results from arrested development and overly protective mothers and detached fathers can be traced back to followers of Sigmund Freud.

"It's nature." "No, it's nurture." "Wrong again—it's society." "You're all wrong—it's a separation from God (Yahweh, Allah)." None of these is a particularly new response to our question on the origins of sexual orientation. But what has changed is the research we have at hand to examine at least some of the proposed answers.

Now, if our attempt to define what it means to be homosexual or bisexual felt a little like we were in a maze avoiding the road blocks as we sought our point of exit, we might compare our efforts to uncover the origins of sexual orientation to being in the middle of a summer blockbuster. In this movie the dedicated scientists sitting in lab coats looking for genetic markers, tracking family histories, or carving up cadavers could easily take on the personas of swashbuckling, high-stakes adventurers: Robert Langdon from *Da Vinci Code* meets Laura Croft from *Tomb Raiders,* a dynamic duo wandering the globe in search of the Book of Origins, a long lost sacred text that details the code of life and human sexuality. And as in every good summer classic, our adventurers are counterbalanced by a group of competitors in the global search—the men and women who are equally determined to carry the message that God and psychology have passed down to them over the ages.

As is standard fare in these summer flicks, we already have the mandatory fighting hordes at war with each other. There are the different factions within the homosexual community and the different coalitions of the religious faithful who are fiercely fighting against gay rights. There is a band of nomadic queer theorists ("you can't oppress me through your manmade heterosexist labels") shooting flaming arrows at the Brotherhood of Gay Essentialist (the "it's biology" group), while a clan of lesbian deconstructionists ("I will not be confined by society's expectations; I am free to create new categories") are hurling spears everywhere, tragically and unintentionally wounding a butch dyke ("I am what I am"). To make the battle even more chaotic, we add in bands of marauding conservative Jews, Christians, and Muslims ("It's a sin against Yahweh or the Trinity or Allah") railing against each other and everyone else on the field, including the moderately religious who are off praying for peace and consensus as well as everyone's soul.

And finally for good measure and to keep everyone horrified, we throw in a plague—let's say AIDS. After all, we have to outdo the rats and beetles that are crawling all over everyone in the other summer adventure film playing in the theater opposite us. Now do we or don't we have the makings of a summer hit?

Too farfetched a story, you say; who will believe it? Well, take away a little hyperbole and the "lights, cameras, roll 'em," and our scripted plot is not far from the truth. Instead of traveling the earth looking for pages from an ancient text, our scientists are studying ancient and contemporary civilizations, using technologies to decipher parts of the human genome, and employing a host of research models to discover the secrets of our origins written into the earth's past and into our cells. And their hard work is yielding results, albeit still preliminary results. And all of this is going on while we are subjected to a cacophony of differing voices, each vying to win the public relations war over how sexual orientation should be viewed and "handled" in the culture.

COMPETING STORIES

Much like the confusion Croft and Langdon might face when they first come across a few pages from the Book of Origins, in real life our research data leave us with incomplete answers and competing stories as we try to answer our question on the origins of sexual orientation. And these competing and, at times, conflicting stories can leave us confused and bewildered. Yet in spite of the contradictions, pieces of the answer are emerging. But putting the pieces together is going to demand time and caution in interpreting the data.

In 1962, Irving Bieber and his team were heralded by many members of the psychiatric community as identifying the cause of homosexuality. Based on a survey of colleagues from across the country, these researchers asserted that they had documented a cause-effect relationship with poor father–son relationships leading to the son's homosexuality.[1] They also suggested that by eliminating these parenting patterns or offering intensive therapy to the adult homosexual, we could prevent or correct the "problem."

By 1973, the tides had changed, and Bieber's professional peers were voting to eliminate homosexuality as a clinical diagnosis and asking serious questions about Bieber's and similar works: Did the supposed pattern found between homosexuality and a sense of isolation or separation from the father figure mean that separation/isolation caused homosexuality? Would it not be just as likely that the child's homosexuality caused the father to withdraw from his son as opposed to the withdrawal causing the homosexuality? And given that the 106 homosexual men used in Bieber's study were under psychiatric care, was it fair and scientifically justifiable to generalize any findings from this group to homosexual men who were not under treatment and living balanced and productive lives? When the American Psychiatric Association (APA) voted to remove homosexuality as a clinical condition, it was a strong rebuke of Bieber's research.

When the APA took these actions, the gay and lesbian community celebrated the victory. At the same time, opponents of the emerging gay rights movement began to look for new ways to fight the threat of this increasingly vocal challenge to what they perceived as American morality. And the public relations wars began.

Twenty years later, in 1993, Dean Hammer[2] and his team at the National Institutes for Health became heroes to many in the gay community. According to some overzealous reporting about his and his team's research, Hamer had identified *the* gay gene. It was located on the X chromosome and was transmitted from mother to son. "We finally have the proof; just as we suspected, sexual orientation is genetic!" cheered homosexuals from across the world. "Foul," yelled the opposition, "just look at Rice's failure to replicate these findings,[3] and if it were genetic, why do we find identical (monozygotic) twins in which one twin is homosexual and the other is heterosexual? Impossible, it can't be genetics!"

With each point and counterpoint, the flames of disagreement that were started years ago grew into an even bigger fire, sometimes stoked by a fresh breeze of new information, but more often by blasts of hot air coming from all sides.

Decades later, some of us are still citing Bieber's research as proof positive of the poor parenting being the cause of homosexuality, while for others of us "the one and only gay gene" is fact certain. Public reactions in these two instances illustrate clearly that as proponents of a particular point of view, we will continue to overstate the findings or accept highly suspect research as clear scientific documentation if the so-called science fits our bias. This should come as no surprise. After all, the Fair Education Foundation, an ultraconservative branch of the creationists' movement, still contends that the sun revolves around the earth and that it can be scientifically proven.

Nonetheless and notwithstanding the exaggerations drawn from some promising research and the continued use of poorly conducted studies, credible science has provided an emerging and growing, if yet incomplete, basis for examining our queer question: What allows Jane to love John, while Betty loves Barb, and Craig would be happy to be with Christine or Christopher? And a good place to start learning about this research is by looking at our furry, feathery, and scaly friends.

YOU'RE SUCH AN ANIMAL

I can see it now: as the credits roll, the first scenes for our summer blockbuster consist of a montage of a day in the life of the Africa jungle and savannah, contrasted against a day in the life of San Francisco and St. Tropez, animals and humans going about their daily routines—hunting, working, eating, grooming, mating, and taking care of their young. And as we pan across wild critters engaging in sex, we dissolve into a close-up of two female bonobos enthralled in mutual masturbation followed by a shot of two male gorillas in the heat of their own sexual activities: another typical day on the planet Earth.

Although long ignored and misinterpreted by biologists, zoologists, and animal anthropologists, sexual encounters among same-sex animals have been going on for a long time on this planet, most probably starting well before humans walked the face of the earth. And these behaviors have much to teach us about our own species.

Our first records of these behaviors among nonhumans date back 2,300 years ago in the form of notes in which Aristotle described the sexual lives of hyenas. Unfortunately, the typically astute Aristotle confused the genitalia of the hyenas, thinking the clitoris was a penis and the labia were a scrotum, but nonetheless, he came to the right conclusion—some of the hyenas he was observing were engaged in same-sex behavior. It just wasn't boy-on-boy hyena sex he was watching; instead it was girl-on-girl hyena sex. Considering the times, it's quite possible that Aristotle was a bit misogynistic in the way he viewed the world.

Until recently, however, most writers who followed Aristotle have ignored these same-gender encounters between animals, or they have explained them away as abhorrent manifestations of aggression instead of acknowledging them as expressions of sexual interest. After all, admitting to themselves that they had seen these behaviors and that the acts appeared to be sexually motivated would have meant raising questions about a fundamental belief about this supposed sin against nature.

I still cringe at the memory of seeing old D-ram mount S-ram repeatedly. . . . True to form and incapable of absorbing this realization at once, I called these actions of the rams "aggressosexual" behavior, for to state that the males had evolved a homosexual society was emotionally beyond me. To conceive of those magnificent beasts as queers—Oh my God! . . . Eventually I called a spade a spade and admitted that rams lived in an essentially homosexual society.

—Valerius Geist 1975, as quoted in Bagemihl 1999, 107

The 1980 writings of T. L. Maple describing orangutan behavior give us an interesting insight into how humans, even so-called scientists, can rationalize what they see and make it fit their own biases: "two male [orangutans] (Dinding and Durian) regularly mouthed the penis of the other on a reciprocal basis. This behavior however, may be nutritively rather than sexually motivated" (Bagemihil 1999, 115). We have to wonder what nutritional value Maple was ascribing to the orangutan semen.

Luckily, with today's expanding conversations on the nature of homosexual behavior in humans, the scientific literature has become more open to exploring and reporting same-sex activities within differing animal species.[4] As examples of this new openness, Bruce Bagemihl (1999) and coauthors Volker Sommer and Paul Vasey (2006) have provided us with two seminal reviews of contemporary and extant literature on same-sex behaviors in nonhuman species ranging from butterflies to whales and apes to zebras. As documented in these texts, the nature of the behaviors vary along different continua similar to the continua that occur among humans, running the gamut from same-sex ritualistic greetings unrelated to sexual attraction to lifelong, same-sex partnering and from the playful sexual interactions among immature members of a species to same-sex intercourse between older members within a social group. It's not only the young engaging in same-sex activities; the silverbacks are doing it too.

In looking at these various displays of same-sex behaviors, it becomes apparent that we can discover much about the origins of similar behaviors within our own species. For example, the ritualized touching of each other's genitals found among male baboons, which appears to have more to do with pledging to act as a cooperative group than with sexual gratification or sexual attraction, is analogous to rituals in which aboriginal groups in Australia touch each other's penises as part of an oath-taking ceremony.[5] These ritual behaviors also correspond to those noted in a reference to oath taking found in Genesis 24:9: "So the servant put his hand between the thighs of Abram, his master, and made a vow to do what Abram asked."

Although these ritualized behaviors appear to be unrelated to sexual gratification or attraction, most other same-gender behaviors among nonhumans seem to be direct expressions of one or both: courtship routines, same-sex copulation with orgasm, same-sex genital masturbation, and the formation of lifelong same-sex couples. Many of the same-sex courtship rituals found within different species are identical to those used in female–male courtship within the species: one sage grouse dances for his male partner as his brother dances for his female partner, an Asian monkey's rear-end flirtations with his latest boyfriend, a hoary marmot's nibbling on her female partner's ear, the bellows from one female koala to another, and the full-mouth kisses with a little tongue action among bonobos—a rather randy group of primates. In most instances, these acts serve as a precursor to sexual interaction—the nonhuman versions of our flirting at the singles' bar and foreplay on the couch before moving into the bedroom.[6]

Researchers have documented other affectionate same-sex interchanges in numbers of species, including some who would be shopping at the big and tall store: gray whales, African elephants, and giraffes. These affectionate behaviors extend from grooming among female gorillas to belly and penis rubbing among gray whales to head rubbing and sexual moaning among male lions to necking among male giraffes (literally rubbing their long necks together while they lick and sniff each other, including their genitals). Such behaviors are frequently precursors to or occur simultaneously with full sexual engagement, including masturbation (e.g., female orangutans, gorillas, and dolphins), fellatio (e.g., macaques), cunnilingus (e.g., hedgehogs), and male-on-male anal penetration (e.g., rams and American bison).[7] You know, if my sweet, old-world mother were alive today, she would probably insist I wash my hands out with soap for typing these words.

At times, the form of sexual engagement is unique to same-gender parings and doesn't follow typical patterns found in opposite-sex behaviors (i.e., the front-to-rear mounting seen in most opposite-sex interactions); in other cases the behavior parallels the animal equivalent of the straight, missionary position among humans.

Most of the critters who engage in same-sex interactions move back and forth and to and fro, with opposite-sex and same-sex behaviors occurring concurrently or at different stages in life. Male mountain zebras will engage in same-sex activities for the first three years of life, with opposite-sex mating more likely than not later in life, whereas many male mountain sheep will routinely move back and forth between same-sex and opposite-sex partners throughout their adolescent and adult lives. Animal watchers have also noted examples of exclusive same-sex pairings in several species. And each year this number grows, not because more same-sex animal pairs are "doing it," but because researchers are showing an increased willingness to *out* those who are.

In some cases, same-sex pairs will co-parent, raising young who have been abandoned—the nonhuman equivalent to foster parenting—or raising young who have been kidnapped from other members of the species. In other cases, female same-sex couples raise offspring who result from one or both partners having mated with male members of the species, the animal equivalent to a growing trend among lesbian couples who are getting their male friends to donate sperm as seed to help create a family. This occurs more frequently among female-dyads and among birds, but there are nonetheless examples of these co-parenting practices among males of various spots and stripes as well, including, on rare occasions, mammals such as male cheetahs.[8]

For some young animals, there are advantages to being raised by two dads or two moms. Chicks being raised by two black male swans are likely to live in top-flight neighborhoods. Their two dads' combined strength and aggression mean the chicks get to live in the big house with the great view.

The literature reports similar parenting patterns among us humans, suggesting that we may have taken a page or two from the nonhuman family-planning texts: Lesbian couples are more likely to raise children than their gay male counterparts. These children may be from prior marriages, the result of sperm donation, adopted, or placed in the home under foster care arrangements.[9]

Roy and Silo, two male chinstrap penguins at the Central Park Zoo, provided possibly the most famous example of a same-sex couple among nonhumans. Living and having sex together for over six years and having made several attempts to incubate rocks, these two penguins incubated an abandoned egg and raised a young female hatchling the zookeeper named Tango—Roy and Silo became national gay figures (Smith 2007).

But alas, in 2005 Silo proved that chinstrap penguins could also be bisexual when he took up with Scrappy, a young female penguin who was brought into the zoo when the exhibit was rearranged (Musbach 2005).

Although we have no current information on whether Roy is using the city of New York's domestic partner benefits with another strapping chinstrap, we do know that the children's story *And Tango Makes Three,* Roy and Silo's story, has been banned in many school libraries. At the same time, these same libraries are placing numbers of books that feature penguins and their heterosexual families on the shelves.

Although same-sex co-parenting is more common among females, same-gender sexual encounters are more common among males than females across most species, including humans. There are, however, some species where females display more frequent same-gender sexual behaviors, as in the case of silver gulls.[10]

For species such as bison and bottlenose dolphins, we observe more same-sex behavior among immature animals who are beginning to experiment with their sexuality,[11] whereas for other animals, such as greylag geese, same-sex behaviors are more common among mature individuals who may have left or lost heterosexual mates.[12] In still other families, as with male gorillas, same-sex pairing will occur across generational lines.[13] The sexual experimentation among immature members of a given species may not be all that different from the same-sex activities noted among adolescents of our own species.[14] Similarly, cross-generational pairing was widely idealized in early Greece.[15]

In studying same-sex behaviors in nature, we find that there are many cases where these behaviors are common in single-sex living groups (the all-boys or all-girls school in the wild as it were), but even more such cases show up in groups where both genders live together. Researchers also note that among most species,[16] same-gender couples don't lose any status within their communities and, in fact, these couples may include community members with the highest social status. And contrary to some assertions that the mounter–mountee relationship is based on dominance, for many of the earth's non-human inhabitants, such as among female Japanese macaques and male common chimpanzees, rank in the social order fails to predict sexual position for same-sex partners. The smaller or younger guy or gal may be on top.

As noted before, same-sex behaviors among nonhumans have striking similarities to human same-sex behaviors. We find young males separated from the rest of the group engaging in same-sex behaviors that would seem to be a form of experimentation and rehearsal for adulthood. We find animals who move back and forth between the genders. There are examples of dominance and submission alongside examples of mutual encouragement, coupled with affection. We see animals who will easily move from one partner to the next and partners who establish long-term relationships. There are female couples who bond to raise their offspring, but never engage in sex with each other, as well as same-gender couples where childrearing and physical affection go hand-in-hand.

If we could apply labels such as homosexuality and bisexuality to animals, we certainly wouldn't do so in every case of same-sex behavior, but there are many examples where we might choose these terms. Some scientists estimate that we would be using these terms in 2 to 6 percent of the animal population—numbers that look very familiar.

IS IT SEX OR AGGRESSION?

When we look at this growing body of literature on same-sex behaviors among animals, some among us question whether the data actually prove that these behaviors are anything more than occasional and strange acts. Other critics suggest that the researchers don't understand what they are seeing: "Those biologists are confusing the drive for dominance with the sex drive." And then there are some of us who will say that even if it is natural for animals to engage in same-sex behaviors, "natural" doesn't mean acceptable or good. Animals also engage in infanticide—would we want people to follow that course?

This resistance to the research and the interpretation of the findings isn't surprising. We understand that if the results and conclusions are accurate and become generally known, this information might lead to a greater acceptance of the same-sex behaviors within the human species. If college or high school biology students learned that boy animals can do it with boy animals and girl animals can do it with girl animals, Jessica and Assad might be more self-accepting when they begin to recognize these same-sex attractions in themselves. And Morey and Susan might view their classmates Jessica and Assad with no, or at least less, disdain if Morey and Susan knew that the king of the jungle at times plays the role of the queen of the jungle, walking off for an afternoon romp in the sand with his boyfriend. Depending on our perspective, this is important or dangerous research—because it begins to normalize homosexuality.

What can be confusing when we look at these criticisms is that some individuals will offer all three at the same time,[17] despite the fact that the first explanation ("it's an aberration and not a natural occurrence") directly conflicts with the other two: "Yes, it occurs in nature, but we don't understand the motivation for the two male chimps masturbating each other," and "Yes,

Bonobos (sometimes referred to as pigmy chimps) could be the poster kids for "Make Love not War." Unlike their cousins the common chimpanzees, who are apt to fight when confronted by another chimp from outside the family, bonobos will use sex to resolve conflict within the family group or with the neighbors from the next village. They build community, in part, through sexual interactions, including same-sex behaviors: female with female and male with male. When they do fight, make-up sex is common after the tiff. These primates also engage in acts that most of us would label as altruistic, compassionate, and empathetic if carried out by humans (Furth and Hoffman 2006).

In some ways, the bonobo village looks like the idealized and, more often than not, unrealized community the 1960s free-love crowd tried to build.

These little primates are among our closest evolutionary relatives. We got the language, but it appears they got the love and peace.

same-sex behavior occurs in nature, but so does cannibalism—are we going to condone both of these despicable behaviors?"

Our first argument raises the question of whether same-sex behaviors occur frequently enough to be seen as more than rare anomalies. Current literature provides plenty of documentation of rates of same-sex behaviors that leave no doubt that these are routinely occurring behaviors. In one study in which the frequency of same-sex behavior was recorded, B. Furth and G. Hoffman[18] found that 55 percent of the sexual encounters involving female bonobos occurred with another female. J. Mann reported even higher rates of same-sex activities among young male bottlenose dolphins.[19] In Paul Vasey's study of Japanese macaques, he recorded seeing all but two of the 16 females under study engage in same-sex activity.[20] The numbers are clear and unequivocal—same-sex behavior is not an anomaly but rather woven into the fabric of animal sexuality. We may have ignored or been unwilling to see it, but it has always been a part of the action in the kingdom. When we look across the more than 500 species researchers have so far identified as exhibiting same-sex behaviors, the numbers of animals who participate in these behaviors track closely to the rates found within humans.

In light of the ever-building evidence, the best educated of our naysayers have begun to alter the arguments. "Yes, we understand the behaviors exist, but you are misinterpreting their underlying meaning" or "Just because these behaviors exist, that doesn't make them right."

Antonio Pardo gives voice to the second argument:

The reproductive instinct of an animal is always directed toward the opposite sex. Therefore an animal can never be homosexual as such the interactions of other instincts (*particularly dominance*) can result in behavior that appears to be homosexual. Such behavior cannot be equated with homosexuality. All it means is that animal sexuality encompasses aspects beyond reproduction.

—As quoted in TFP Committee on American Issues 2004, p. 93

Those critics who argue that researchers are misinterpreting same-gender behaviors as sexually motivated also assert an interesting and somewhat bewildering presupposition that only behaviors that can lead to procreation can be used to define an animal's sexual proclivities. Because same-gender acts can't lead to procreation, they must serve another purpose, a purpose unrelated to the animal's sexual drive. These behaviors must be acts of aggression, efforts to prove dominance or attempts to curry favor from a superior; they have nothing to do with affection or sexual attraction. It's easy to see how this argument fits certain acts in which humans engage. Rape in the jail cell doesn't speak about sexual preference.[21] But jailhouse rapes and other acts of asserting dominance do not even come close to accounting for the majority of same-sex acts in humans or in nonhuman species.

The assertions presented in this argument are flawed in several different ways. In assuming that opposite-sex encounters are motivated solely by the desire to procreate, the argument ignores evidence that same-sex and opposite-sex nonhuman partners establish long-term and lifelong sexual relationships (e.g., black-wing stilts, ocellated antbirds, herring gulls, red-backed shrikes, kittiwakes, Humboldt penguins) and that these relationships continue after procreation ceases (e.g., killer whales, Canada Geese, and oystercatchers).[22] Sex doesn't necessarily end when procreation stops.

This argument also fails to account for the data collected for several species showing that there is no apparent relationship between the active versus passive role during sex and the dominant and submissive roles during other day-to-day activities.[23] Same-sex encounters among animals also include activities where neither partner can be labeled as the dominant or aggressive partner: mutual masturbation and mutual cunnilingus. When Hilda and Heidi the hedgehogs were engaged in mutual cunnilingus, it really looked like it was about sexual gratification to me. The same is true when Roger and Rodney, two male rams, took turns backing up to one another, each encouraging his friend to engage him in penile-to-anal intercourse.

The third argument links same-sex behavior with infanticide, insisting that both are evils that may occur in nature but that neither can be tolerated among humans. This argument proposes, "Some animals engage in infanticide, and some animals engage in same-sex behavior. Infanticide is wrong; therefore, same-sex behavior must be wrong for humans."

When this argument is offered, there is never any evidence or even suggestion that the same animals are engaging in both behaviors. Those who offer this argument don't even suggest that infanticide occurs in all or even most of the species where same-sex behavior can be found. Nor is there any explanation of how or why the two actions are related except to attest that if you accept that humans should not participate in infanticide, a proposition almost all of us would accept, then you must accept that humans should not participate in same-sex behavior.

The only correlation I have been able to find is that those who make this argument find both same-sex behavior and infanticide deplorable, making them somehow related. Interestingly enough, most instances of infanticide are motivated by the male animal's desire to breed with the mother of the offspring he has killed—the desire to procreate.

For those who are inclined to reject same-sex behavior as a part of nature or see it as a negative part of nature, one or all of these three arguments are likely to resonate. For those of us who think same-sex behaviors are a part of nature and either are neutral in value or should be celebrated as part of human diversity, the innumerable documented observations of same-sex behaviors across animal species are likely to resonate.

The growing weight of the evidence is unquestionably on the side of those arguments that accept that same-sex behaviors occur throughout the animal kingdom, including humans. But of course, the question of the value placed on these behaviors is certainly up for discussion. I suspect that if and when these data are included in the general biology textbooks, the argument that asserts same-sex behaviors are rare anomalies will be difficult to sustain. What we have to wonder is, how long will it take us to get the information into the texts, and how strong will the political pressure be to hide the science?

TWO NON-BIOLOGICAL THEORIES

Before moving on to talk about the biology of sexual orientation in humans, this is probably a good place to pause and introduce two alternative answers to our question about why Betty is so attracted to Barb. The two theories we are going to look at are offered by individuals who stand at polar opposites when it comes to all things homosexual, except for the fact that proponents of both propositions disagree that homosexuality is either an essential or an immutable element in a person's identity. On one side of the debate, we hear the voices that point to deficit parenting and not biology as the cause of homosexuality. On the other side, we hear the arguments of queer theorists who believe that homosexuality is a manmade construct, a term coined by society to isolate people who choose to engage in particular actions that are part of a natural array of behaviors, behaviors that should not be used to define or separate people into neat little categories.

Although we begin our discussion on both theories here, the research on deficit parenting will receive closer attention in the chapter on reparative therapy and ex-gay ministries. Queer theory is addressed to a lesser degree in chapter 6, "The Downfall of Society," which talks about the history of homosexuality, and in the chapter 8, on the "secret homosexual agenda."

Deficit Parenting and a Loving Father

The year I turned 50, my mother told me that she and my father should have known that I was gay when I was three. In retrospect, the differences between my brother Stan and me were so stark that she now couldn't imagine how she and Dad had failed to piece things together well before I was 17 and came out to the two of them—a coming-out that was prompted by a direct question from Dad.

I was five or six years old when an older cousin who grew up in the small town where my Dad had been raised came to visit. At that time, he was a member of the Marine Corps' Presidential Honor Guard and the most amazing-looking man I had ever seen, tall, handsome, and with a smile that could melt an iceberg. I certainly didn't understand it then, but this was my first crush. When he arrived, he brought me a toy space helmet, which I wore every day and all day for weeks. My brother Stan and I both thought Joe was great. Stan wanted to follow in Joe's footsteps; I wanted to follow Joe home.

As time went on, the difference between my parents' two sons became ever more apparent. Stan played football, ran track, and did one heck of a job on the lawn. I, on the other hand, would go off on Saturdays to debate tournaments, took roles in school plays, and butchered the yard. Stan still contends I did a poor job mowing the lawn so that Dad would keep it as a Stan chore. Stan developed crushes on our older sister's girlfriends. I developed crushes on Stan's boyfriends. He was taller; I was shorter.

Despite these differences, one thing Stan and I had in common was the attention we got from our father. Although Dad was reserved in most public displays of affection, there was no doubt in either Stan's or my mind that Dad loved us deeply. He proudly went to Stan's Friday night football games, ending up on the field when Stan was hurt. On Saturdays he would show up at my debate tournaments, smiling from ear to ear when I won and being extremely supportive when I didn't. He read to us as children and made snow sculptures for us in the winter. Other kids had snowmen; we had snow rabbits, snow horses, and any number of other snow animals in our yard. In the winter, Dad also took his two sons and two daughters to the local skating rink and helped us learn how to maneuver around the ice, encouraging all four of us to move at our own pace; mine was slower than Stan's, but it didn't seem to matter to Dad. He knew I was a klutz; it was just who I was— his uncoordinated younger son whom he loved. On Sunday evenings in the summer, my siblings and I climbed into the family car with both parents, stopped to get ice cream cones, and parked by the fence at a local baseball field, watching two local teams play each other. Stan watched the game; I sat soaking up the warmth of our family being together. I'm not sure what my two sisters were thinking about, but this was a family connected by love and the occasional childish outburst: "I get to sit up front this time!"

In my entire life, the only time I saw Dad's affection for me change was shortly after he asked me if I was homosexual and I said yes. After a few weeks of pandemonium around our house—Mom and Dad did not take my coming-out well—I noticed a shift in Dad's behavior. He moved even closer to me. Although this change in behavior was obvious to me and helped off-set Mom's crying spasms, I never really thought much about the change. Ours was a very conservative, church- and family-centered home. I also noticed that Dad, in his usual style, was reading, but the topic of the books shifted. Now the books were on homosexuality.

I was, of course, too self-absorbed to stop and ask what was in those books. As far as I was concerned, Dad just liked to read on any topic that came up. Years later, I discovered what was in those books. Dad was reading such books as George Henry's *Sex Variants: A Study of Homosexual Patterns* and Irving Bieber's *Homosexuality: A Psychoanalytic Study.* And in these texts, he was reading passages such as Bieber's unequivocal statement: "In my long experience, I have not found a single case where, in the developing years, a father had a kind, affectionate, and constructive relationship with the son who becomes homosexual. This has been an unvarying finding. . . . if a father has a kind, affectionate, and constructive relationship with his son, he will not produce a homosexual son."[24] And in Henry's work, he was reading case histories of homosexual men and women, each somewhat different, but nonetheless each with a pattern of a dysfunctional family.[25]

One other change that occurred when my parents made me fully open the closet door, which I had been leaving somewhat ajar, was that I started seeing a local psychiatrist, who I don't think was following a therapy protocol of which my parents, or at least my mother, would have approved. Dr. Sprague was trying to help me understand how I was going to have to adapt to society and my parents and how I was going to handle my own internalized homophobia (a term that wasn't coined at the time I was seeing Dr. Sprague). He and I also talked about how I was going to need to help my parents accept who I was. There was never any mention of a "cure." I don't think Dr. Sprague believed I needed to be or could be cured. For me, he was the perfect shrink, one who was a decade ahead of the APA.

Years later, as I reflected on what had happened during the time of my coming-out, I began to examine different pieces of the picture. Some of these pieces still bring me joy. My parents had shown such love for their children that I knew I could tell them that I was gay and even be obnoxious about it at various times, and I had nothing to fear. I was their son, and they weren't going to leave me out in the cold. They would be by my side, loving me into and through adulthood. Of course, I am sure my mother prayed until the day she died that I would find a woman who would convince me I had made a mistake. In looking at the picture in its totality and from the vantage point provided by time, I also saw elements that brought me great sadness, one being that Dad had read those books.

What Dad was reading were the texts that would eventually serve as a foundation for reparative therapy (see chapter 5, "Reparative Therapy and the Ex-Gay Identity," in this book). He was reading that my homosexuality could be traced to a failure on his part to develop a healthy relationship with me. He was being told that children have basic identity needs that can be satisfied only by the same-gender parent, and if these needs are not met as the child approaches puberty, she or he will sexualize the unmet needs, eventually trying to fulfill them in relationships with same-gender partners.[26] Those books were trying to convince him that I was looking for the relationship that I didn't have with him and seeking it in the men I was seeing.

As evidence of an underlying disruption in the father–son or mother–daughter relationship, members of NARTH (the National Association for Research & Therapy of Homosexuality) point to personal testimonies from individuals who have sought therapy to change their sexual orientation and to Irving Bieber's 1962 survey of therapists who engaged in psychoanalytic therapy with homosexuals.[27] What I don't know, because I hadn't stopped to really look at the picture until after Dad's death, was whether he realized that evidence offered in support of a deficit parenting model was terribly flawed. (Again, see chapter 5.) Drawing cause-effect relationships from these data was highly suspect. When a father distances himself from a son who exhibits atypical male characteristics, it could be that the homosexuality caused the non-masculine characteristics, and these characteristics in turn led to the separation with the father.[28] So the real question at hand was, had these sons developed what was perceived as non-heterosexual behaviors because their fathers separated themselves from their sons, or did some fathers estrange themselves from their sons because the sons showed non-heterosexual behaviors? And what accounts for the homosexuality in sons who had strong and healthy relationships with their fathers?

In studying relationships between fathers and sons, Kory Floyd and his colleagues helped provide part of the answer to the question of which came first. In their study, this team looked at the reported affection shown by fathers of four different groups: (1) heterosexual sons, (2) homosexual sons whose fathers didn't know their sons were homosexual, (3) homosexual sons whose fathers were unsure whether their sons were or were not homosexual, and (4) homosexual sons whose fathers were fully aware of their sons' homosexuality. When these researchers looked at the data, they found, as predicted, that overall, homosexual sons received fewer signs of affection from their fathers than heterosexual sons, a finding that is certainly consistent with the deficit parenting model. But when they separated out the three groups of homosexual sons, they found that sons whose fathers didn't know about their sexual orientation received the highest levels of affection of any of the groups, including the heterosexual sons. Lack of affection didn't cause homosexuality; it was more likely that the father's recognition that his son was homosexual caused him to withdraw, possibly out of fear, distain, or uncertainty about how to interact. Which came first, the rooster or the egg? It was the egg—the sons' homosexuality preceded the fathers' behavior.

As in all such studies, there are cases that don't conform to the results for the group as a whole. I was one of those lucky eggs. When Dad put two and two together, he didn't withdraw; rather, he moved closer—he was going to make sure that I knew he loved me. Now that I more fully understand the change in his behavior, I wish that I could have told him that I loved the additional attention, the jokes, and so on, but that there was never a day in my life when I didn't know that he loved me, nor was there a day in my life when I thought he treated me more harshly or with less caring than he treated Stan. Actually, to me and to my brother, it seemed that I got treated better in most situations.

I hope that Dad was able to heal or rise above whatever damage might have resulted to his sense of self from reading that awful literature. He deserved to know that he was a great dad before he asked me to step out of the closet as well as after I stepped out. I have a number of friends who talk about the difficulties that they had with their fathers, but I also know those who had experiences similar to mine. I raise my glass in a toast to all of those dads: W. D., Dennis, Larry, Chuck, Raymond, Walter, and Stan Sr., I salute and thank you. We are better men because you were our fathers.

Queer Theory

In the 1990s, queer theorists told us that there were no homosexuals; at least there were none until we labeled them as such in the 1890s.[29] Strongly influenced by philosopher Michel Foucault, lesbian feminism, and the social constructionist movement, queer theory proposed that before we created the label, there were no homosexuals; all we had were people who engaged in different forms of same-sex behaviors. In some societies these behaviors were condemned and punished; in some societies these behaviors were accepted and even honored. But in both sets of societies, the actions didn't define the person. People weren't divided into homosexuals and heterosexuals or into homosexuals, bisexuals, and heterosexuals. They were just people who did or did not engage in specific behaviors.

If we looked across cultures, we could find preadolescent Sambian males from New Guinea regularly ingesting the semen of their adolescent peers. The preadolescent was expect to swallow the sperm as nourishment for his maturation into manhood, while his adolescent brother or cousin was ejaculating in preparation for his eventual heterosexual marriage. Within indigenous American cultures, we had some adult males dressing as women and living as the wives of young hunters. And in the late 1800s, two middle-class American women might live together in what was referred to as a Boston marriage, an intimate partnership without overtly acknowledged sex.[30] Each of the groups displayed very different behavior patterns that meant very different things within their cultures.

According to queer theory, similar same-sex pairings have been a part of the human repertoire of behaviors practiced throughout history, but none of these people were "homosexuals," at least not until the late 19th and early 20th centuries when we constructed the word *homosexual*. Bothered by same-sex behaviors, our culture chose to group everyone who engaged in these various practices into one cluster, place a medical label on the members of this group, and declare their behaviors as immutable or essential parts of their beings.

As evidence for their social constructionist argument, queer theorists point to cultures where same-sex behaviors were openly practiced but where there were no words for homosexuality or for heterosexuality. In Ancient Greece it wasn't the gender of the person with whom a man slept that determined how he was judged; it was the position the man assumed during sex that placed him into the good or bad category, in this case superior versus subordinate. If the man was the active partner (he who inserts his penis), he demonstrated his superior social status. If he was the passive partner (the person who is penetrated), he was considered the subordinate—a position appropriately filled by young men, women, slaves, and foreigners, but one that could bring derision if assumed by an adult male citizen.[31] The Greeks didn't create a system to divide people based on sexual orientation; they chose to divide men based on gender expression or power relationships and more often than not to ignore women. Other societies could presumably divide people based on other characteristics: Does the individual prefer certain sexual acts? Does the individual engage in specific fetishes?

According to queer theorists, yes, some of us do engage in same-sex intimacy, but this is not an innate or immutable characteristic of our very essence. People can and do move back and forth between the sexes when picking intimate partners. There is nothing wrong with same-sex behaviors, but should we engage in these actions, we need to avoid identifying ourselves as homosexuals or gays or lesbians. Instead, we need to join together with other disenfranchised (queer) groups, including prostitutes and individuals who practice sadism and masochism, to exert our freedom. Dividing people into these different categories serves no purpose except to control and limit.

The behaviors that underlie the constructs of heterosexuality and homosexuality aren't central to our being, but when we apply these labels to ourselves, we segregate into socially defined classes of normal versus deviant or deficient—social classes that can and will vary within and across cultures. If we were a male of 30 in any number of cultures, there would have been nothing wrong with marrying a 15-year-old girl. Of course, in today's Western culture, these acts would be sufficient reason for us to hide in the shadows of society and vey possibly end up in jail. At least some queer theorists would argue that no such judgments should be made based on these or any number of other sexual behaviors, nor should we classify an individual as anything except human based on these behaviors. (The acceptance of these behaviors raises serious issues regarding exploitation, coercion, and the use power in sexual practices. For further discussion, see chapters 7 and 8.)

For the queer theorist, the origin of homosexuality is not biology or bad parenting; the origin lies in society's decision to construct and use the word *homosexual*. In response to that choice, the queer theorist reclaims the word *queer* and asserts that all humans who fall under this expanding umbrella (e.g., lesbians, gay men, intersex individuals, transgendered persons, prostitutes, persons who practice bondage, etc.) should stop trying to assimilate into the culture. Instead, we must reconstruct the culture to accept individuals as they present themselves without the use of labels.

A recent survey conducted by Hunter College found that only 13 of over 700 nonheterosexual respondents had adopted the label "queer" in describing themselves (Egan, Edelman, and Sherrill 2008).

In responding to queer theorists, writers such as Boswell, Holland, and Hubbard argue that drawing distinctions between persons based on the sex of their intimate partners is not unique to current Western culture but rather has occurred throughout history. Even in those cultures where we don't find words for homosexuality or heterosexuality, the literature gives detailed descriptions of individuals who are exclusive in their preferences for same-sex partners, and it provides clear examples of same-sex cohorts banding together as a subgroup within the larger community: for example, the Sacred Band of Thebes—a fierce troop of fourth-century B.C.E. Greek soldiers composed of male lovers—and the Molly houses of England, 18th-century taverns in England where men who engaged in same-sex behaviors would gather to socialize and hook up. Although the Greeks may not have had terms equivalent to *homosexual* or *heterosexual,* they offered myths and other dialogues as explanations for the differences among men and women who slept exclusively with same-gender partners and those who preferred opposite-gender partners.[32] Homosexuality, bisexuality, and heterosexuality may have gone unnamed in some societies, but these different attributes did not go without notice or comment throughout history.

When we consider the central question of whether homosexuality is an innate characteristic or a social construct, we find cases for both answers. Certainly not all same-sex behaviors could or should be used to classify someone as homosexual, but throughout time there have been people, women and men, who have been singularly physically and emotionally attracted to members of the same sex. Although we would easily exclude preadolescents and adolescents participating in the Sambian coming-of-age rituals as fitting our definition of homosexuality, some of these young men grew up to live with each other instead of entering into heterosexual marriage.[33] There have always been individuals who fit our definition of homosexual even when there was no word *homosexual.*

In looking at the research on sexual behaviors among animals, we find that many of these practices are quite consistent with queer theory—for example, the free-flowing movement from opposite-gender to same-gender behaviors among the bonobos.[34] But there are some significant findings that challenge the premise that same-sex attraction is not an essential or innate part of individual animals. For example, many rams will engage in same-gender sex when confined to an all-male group. However, when ewes are introduced to the herd, most but not all of these males will begin to engage in opposite-sex mating, becoming exclusively devoted to heterosexual-like behaviors. At the same time, there are some rams who will continue to show no interest in females; their only interest is other rams. And researchers are identifying the physiological traits that differentiate these particular members of the species.[35] It appears that there are rams that are dyed-in-the-wool homosexuals.

Queer theory offers some interesting observations on how culture limits and controls behavior and on how we define ourselves based on repeated behavior patterns and social labels. But as some historians have pointed out, queer theory fails to account for a body of literature that clearly differentiates between people exclusively attracted to same-sex partners and those attracted to opposite-sex partners. Queer theory also fails to account for the growing body of research on the biology of sexual orientation.

BACK TO BIOLOGY

Patterns of homosexuality in family groups (e.g., higher incidence rates of homosexuality among same-sex siblings, in particular among identical twins, and higher rates that follow maternal bloodlines) provide us with some of the strongest evidence that biology plays an important, but not necessarily singular, role in determining an individual's sexual orientation. The presence of a biological link is further supported by the differences in secondary characteristics (differences in brain lateralization, responses to human pheromones, etc.) that we find when comparing homosexual and heterosexual individuals. In exploring which biological factors might play a role in determining sexual orientation, researchers have been looking at genetic links as well as hormonal triggers.

Patterns of Homosexuality within Families

In an effort to understand the role genetics play in the origins of sexual orientation, J. Michael Bailey and his colleagues conducted several studies of twins, both identical (monozygotic) and non-identical (dizygotic), collecting data on their sexual orientation and the sexual orientation of their biological and adopted siblings. In one study focused on female twins,[36] the research group found that if Mary, a female monozygotic (identical) twin, was homosexual, there was a 48 percent chance that her twin sister Mattie would also be homosexual. Carrying this further, if Mary or Mattie was homosexual, there was a 14 percent likelihood that Mavis, a non-twin birth sister, would be homosexual. And finally, if Mary or Mattie was homosexual, there was a 6 percent chance that Marla, an adopted sister, would be homosexual. This pattern demonstrates that if one sibling was homosexual, there was an increased probability that her biological sister would also be homosexual, and if they carried the same exact alleles (identically matched genetic material), as in identical twins, the probability was even higher. However, when there was no blood relationship between adopted sisters who were raised together, the odds returned to rates only slightly higher than those found throughout the culture. These findings were further borne out by the fact that if Susie, a female dizygotic (nonidentical) twin, was homosexual, there was only a 16 percent chance that Sandy, her nonidentical twin, would be homosexual. We find similar concordance rates (i.e., both same-sex siblings being homosexual) for male twins and male non-twins.[37]

In replicating the results of these initial twin studies, Katherine Kirk joined Bailey and his colleagues in conducting a survey of 980 monozygotic and 928 dizygotic sets of twins drawn from the Australian national twin registry.[38] As part of this larger study, the research team was able to calculate estimations of heritability of sexual orientation for the Australian twins. These estimations of heritability tell us how much of the differences in sexual orientation found within a group can be attributed to genetics. Based on the survey results, the researchers estimated that genetics accounted for 50 to 60 percent of the variance in sexual orientation among female monozygotic twins. For identical male twins, genetics accounted for 30 to 45 percent of the variance in sexual orientation.

At the same time that Kirk, Bailey, and their colleagues were conducting research using the twin registry in Australia, Kenneth Kendler and his associates were conducting a similar study as part of a national survey in the United States.[39] When they calculated the heritability estimates for sexual orientation for their sample of 794 pairs of twins, they found that genetic differences accounted for somewhere between 28 and 65 percent of the variability. Kendler's sample did not allow him to calculate separate estimates of heritability for females and males.

These two studies help us to understand the role that genetics plays in determining sexual orientation. It isn't 100 percent of the answer, but genes are certainly a part of the equation. Of course, these results are far from telling us how many genes may be involved or how much influence these genes play in any given person. In considering these studies, it's also important to remember that the results are dependent on accuracy in reporting sexual orientation on the survey. If Tim reports that he is homosexual but his identical twin Tom isn't comfortable with his own sexual orientation and reports that he is heterosexual (as might be expected in at least some cases), we will end up with an underestimation of the influence of genetics.

Critics of biology as part of the equation are likely to ask how if one identical twin is homosexual, the other twin could be anything but homosexual.

After all, don't identical twins have virtually 100 percent concordance for hair and eye color, height, and other basic traits? Although this is almost always true for these particular characteristics, there are a number of genetically linked physical and behavioral traits with much lower concordance rates and heritability estimates among monozygotic (identical) twins: color blindness, brain lateralization in language processing, handedness, differences in dermal ridges in fingerprints, autism, and type 1 insulin-dependent diabetes, to name but a few.[40] These lower concordance rates for monozygotic twins may result from differences in genetics that occur after the fertilized egg splits or from the way genes express themselves because of different pre- or post-birth environments.

Although monozygotic twins begin with the same genetic material, there are times when differences in these genes can occur pre- and post birth. Two causes for these differences are genetic fragility or a recently discovered phenomenon known as CVN (copy number variation).[41] CVN occurs when a particular gene either fails to copy in one of the two twins or when the gene creates two or more copies of itself in one of the twins. Edwards, Dent, and Kahn present an example of what may be the most dramatic type of discordance in monozygotic twins. In one case study, they report on a pair of monozygotic twins who shared the same genetic makeup at conception, but due to a loss of the Y chromosome after the initial cell division, one twin took on a female gender, whereas the other twin remained a male[42]—monozygotic yes, identical no.

Differences in monozygotic twins can also result from various environmental factors found in utero, changing the way a particular gene expresses itself. Maternal hormone levels can impact each twin differently because each lives in his or her own environment in the womb. Identical twins will often be carried in their own individual birth sac (chronic membrane) and possibly in their own placenta. As a result, they may be exposed to different maternal hormone levels. In other cases identical twins who share the same placenta can be positioned so that one twin gets better nourishment. These variations in environment can create differences in the biology of the identical twins. Even if Beauchamp and Beauregard carry the exact same blue blood in their veins, Mom's body may, unwittingly, be playing favorites while the two boys are in the womb. And the differences in the way they are treated in their mother's body may cause variations in their biology, albeit not in their genetics. Monozygotic twins can be less than 100 percent identical.

In addition to documenting that biology plays a role in determining sexual orientation among twins and their siblings, research on patterns within families suggests that in many instances male homosexuality is likely to be carried through the mother's bloodline or pedigree.[43] This pattern of transmission can be traced by following women who have homosexual brothers.

These women have a higher probability of giving birth to homosexual sons than we would expect in the general population. The daughters of these women also have an increased likelihood of having a gay son. This may occur as a result of genes being transmitted by the mother, or it might be related to a mother's inherited tendency to develop immunity to male hormones, which could lead to homosexuality originating during pregnancy. (This possible hormonal link is discussed in a subsequent section in this chapter.) Although this maternal transmission pattern is significant, it certainly does not account for all occurrences of homosexuality, nor does it mean that every boy born to a woman who has a homosexual brother will be born homosexual. If it did, we would have a method for committing homosexual genocide, at least for males, which some fear may prove to be a real threat as we move closer to understanding the biology of sexual orientation.

Thanks, Mom—Love the Genes

Recognizing the influence of genetics and the fact that homosexuality in men often tracks the maternal bloodline, Dean Hamer and his research group at the National Institutes of Health began studying the X chromosomes in brothers who were both homosexual but were not twins.[44] Hamer and colleagues were trying to determine which if any genetic markers on the X chromosome were consistently held in common by homosexual brothers who were assumed to have inherited their predisposition to homosexuality from their mothers. Because these researchers were focused at looking at males who appeared to be homosexual as a result of maternal pedigrees, they excluded brothers where paternal pedigree or male transmission was likely (e.g., if the brothers' father was homosexual or if either of the brothers had a homosexual son of his own). Hamer was studying the influence of mom's genes, not dad's.

As with all males, each of Hamer's brothers had a Y chromosome inherited from his father and an X chromosome inherited from his mother. The genetic makeup on the Y chromosome for both brothers was always the same because Dad has only one Y chromosome to pass on to his sons. If you're a man, and your Y chromosome is a bit wacky, you can blame your dad as well as your paternal granddad and great granddad. In contrast, Mom has two X chromosomes, one she inherited from her mother and one she inherited from her father. This means that the specific X chromosome that Mom passes on to her son would include a split in its genetic composition: on average, one-half of the genes on the son's X chromosome would come from his maternal grandmother, and one-half would come from his maternal grandfather. His brother would also be expected to have an approximate 50/50 split, but not the exact same split as the first brother.

When Hamer compared the genetic markers on the X chromosome from Paul to the markers from brother Peter, he could expect that approximately half of Paul and Peter's DNA markers on this chromosome would be the same, and half of the their DNA markers would be different. Likewise, when Hamer compared brother Romulus to brother Remus, he would expect to find a somewhat different 50/50 split in the brothers' DNA markers. An approximate 50/50 split did occur when comparing the genetic markers in each of the 40 pairs of homosexual brothers, none of whom were monozygotic twins, except for the DNA markers at one site on the X chromosome (Xq28). In 33 (83%) of 40 cases, the genetic marker at Xq28 was the same for both brothers. It would be hard to believe that this was just another random occurrence. Something was going on. In response, Hamer and crew hypothesized that one of the genes located at site Xq28 influenced the sexual orientation in those 33 pairs of brothers. He and his team never attempted to identify the particular gene at this site on the X chromosome that was the hero or culprit, depending on your point of view. Nor did they claim that a single gene on this marker was the sole trigger for male sexual orientation. All they said was that it appeared that one of the genes at the Xq28 marker seemed to contribute to homosexuality when transmitted through the maternal bloodline. To check these results, members of Hamer's NIH team replicated their original findings using 32 additional pairs of twins.[45] They found virtually the same results.

Since Hamer's original study, one other study has examined the genetic marker at Xq28. However, in this study the research team included men with paternal uncles who were homosexual. This meant that Rice and his colleagues were studying homosexuals whose sexual orientation may have originated through their father's gene pool. Not surprisingly, the Xq28 markers in these pairs of brothers did not show an above-normal rate of concordance. Rice and his colleagues' study is often assumed to disprove or call into question Hamer's findings and subsequent hypothesis. Hamer, however, claims that there is no contradiction in the results in the three studies. In his two studies, he and his team were looking at brothers who had maternal pedigrees that included homosexuality, whereas Rice's study included gay brothers with paternal pedigrees for homosexuality. The origins in these different groups should not be expected to be the same, especially if there are multiple biological pathways to sexual orientation. If you were looking for a gene that transmitted homosexuality from a father, you wouldn't be looking at the X chromosome—all of us boys get that one from our moms.

In a study in 2005, Brian Mustanski and Michael DuPree[46] reexamined the DNA samples used in Hamer and Hu's earlier research and added 73 new families with two or more homosexual brothers to the mix. As opposed to focusing exclusive attention on the X chromosome, this group of researchers conducted a full genome scan in an attempt to locate genetic links to male homosexuality. In their study Mustanski and DuPree found possible sites located on three different chromosomes (7, 8, and 9). But as is so often the case, they couldn't point to a specific set of genes. One more time we have strong circumstantial evidence of genetics, but no smoking gun.

Whether we buy the claims that Rice's study disproves Hamer's work, we accept Hamer's explanation that the groups that they studied had different paths of transmission, or we believe that further analyses of chromosomes 7, 8, and 9 or the X chromosome would yield evidence of specific genes that contribute to homosexuality, there are two things that seem certain. First, Hamer did not find, nor did he claim to find, *the* gay gene. Nonetheless, the evidence in total does point to some genetic contributions to sexual orientation. A third thing we know is that when Hamer's research was first published, there were a lot of mothers with homosexual sons who were looking very closely at their brothers, and there were a lot of sisters with homosexual brothers who were looking very closely at their sons.

Hormones

We understand, and often comment about, the effects of hormones during adolescence and the hormonal effects on middle-aged adults: "What do you expect? He's a teenager, and his hormones are raging." "Her estrogen levels are on a seesaw; of course she has mood swings." But hormones play an even more critical role in prenatal and perinatal development and, as such, may prove a key component in the biological origins of sexual orientation. Intrigued by several animal studies showing a link between same-sex behavior and hormones,[47] researchers have examined whether variances in human sexual orientation might also be attributable to differences in prenatal hormone levels—a hypothesis supported by three lines of research.

We can see the dramatic impact of prenatal hormones on sexual orientation in a genetically recessive defect known as congenital adrenal hyperplasia (CAH). In its classic form, CAH causes an overproduction of male hormones in the unborn fetus. When CAH occurs in unborn females, it can cause masculinization of the female genitalia ranging from a mild enlargement of the clitoris to a fully developed penis. If diagnosed in utero, hormone replacement can be used to negate these changes in genitalia. CAH has also been shown to affect sexual orientation in some of these girls, as documented by increased incidences of homosexual fantasies (48%) and same-sex behaviors (22%) in adult women who experienced the disorder. [48]

In the second line of study, researchers have found less physically dramatic effects of prenatal hormones in female children of mothers who took a nonsteroidal hormone known as diethylstilbestrol (DES) during pregnancy. Daughters born to mothers who took this drug, which was prescribed during high-risk pregnancies, have been shown to have an increased attraction to same-sex partners in adulthood. However, unlike with CAH, these women showed no change or masculinization in their genitalia.[49]

Theorists have hypothesized that the pattern of homosexuality among younger brothers may also provide evidence of possible prenatal hormonal influences on sexual orientation. When examining homosexuality among men, Ray Blanchard[50] and others have determined that the greater the number of older brothers a boy has, the higher the likelihood that he will be homosexual. Combining this pattern in birth order with a pattern of lower birth weights in male homosexuals who have older heterosexual bothers, Blanchard and some of his colleagues have theorized that in giving birth to sons, mothers may begin to develop an antibody for male-specific hormones. In subsequent pregnancies, these antibodies could interrupt the flow of male hormones that help organize masculine characteristics in the male fetus, leading to same-sex attraction and other physical characteristics. These theorists further suggest that because individual fetuses may be more or less susceptible to such antibodies, it cannot be assumed that every male child following the first homosexual son would in turn be homosexual, but there is a continued increase likelihood of same-sex sexual orientation. A similar pattern occurs when Rh-negative mothers give birth to both Rh-positive and Rh-negative children depending on the fetus's response to the mother's hormone levels.[51]

Although this antibody theory is consistent with the data on prenatal hormonal differences in females and with different animal studies,[52] opponents of the theory tell us that increased likelihood of second, third, and fourth sons being gay could just as easily be explained by the fact that fathers have less time to pay attention to these late-birth-order sons. This alternative explanation is certainly consistent with the deficit parenting theory we began talking about earlier.

Related Physiological and Neurological Traits

Ask a member of your family or a friend to describe the traits associated with being a lesbian and the traits associated with being a gay male. Then ask the same person to describe the traits associated with being a straight male and those associated with straight women. You are likely to get some pretty interesting and revealing answers, some of which may tell you about the cultural perspectives discussed by queer theorists: for example, masculine vs. effeminate, artistic vs. athletic, tasteful vs. boorish, sleazy vs. moral, open-minded vs. biased, and the list can go on and on and on. Now, if you take the list and try to apply each characteristic to individuals within the four different categories (gay male, straight male, lesbian, straight female), what you will find is that some of the stereotypes do work with some people in the given category. But the same characteristics could also be applied to individuals who fall into any of the other three categories. I am sure that most of us know masculine gay men and masculine lesbians and that we also know masculine straight men and masculine heterosexual women. (Of course some of us may not know that the masculine gay man is in fact gay or that the masculine heterosexual woman is straight.) We also know effeminate gay men as well as effeminate straight men. Every one of these terms fits someone we each know in all four categories, as well as our bisexual friends and acquaintances. But at the same time, some of these characteristics are probably not distributed equally across each category. I confess that sometimes when a characteristic shows up in the often-assumed-wrong category, its appearance confuses me for a minute or two. I remember when I met a friend's

One of the physical traits that has been linked to differences in sexual orientation among women is finger-length ratio for the index (D2) and ring (D4) fingers. When D2 and D4 are similar in length, it is more likely that a woman will be heterosexual, whereas homosexual women's index fingers tend to be shorter than their ring fingers, as are men's. Studying this phenomenon, Lynn Hall and Craig Love (2003) found that when monozygotic twins were discordant for sexual orientation, the heterosexual twin and the homosexual twin would have different finger-length ratios, with the heterosexual sister having little to no difference in the length of the two fingers. When monozygotic twins where concordant for sexual orientation, their finger-length ratios were also concordant.

husband-to-be and marked him down as a gay man in training. Now 30 some years later, I understand how wrong I was. And I am glad that I didn't ask him out; it could have ruined a great friendship. I also remember the dinner party where I met two gay hog farmers. These delightful men caused me to rethink what it meant to be gay. (See chapter 7 for more discussion on stereotyping.)

Although our friends and many of us continue to play games with stereotypes, there are some serious researchers who are exploring a number of other characteristics that may better track sexual orientation. But just as our stereotypes don't fit 100 percent of the time, the characteristics with which these researchers are working also are highly unlikely to be proof positive of a given sexual orientation. After all, few things are absolute within genetic makeup of individuals across a given species. Yes, men are taller as a group than are women. But my friend Lauren, a women's basketball coach, has to sit down to have an eye-to-eye conversation with me. You're right—she is a tall woman, and I am a short man. She is also an attractive heterosexual woman—oh well, there goes one of those stereotypes up in flames.

During their explorations these researchers have documented sets of physical and neurological characteristics that may differentiate gay men as a group from heterosexual men as a group and lesbians from heterosexual women. For example, there is an increased likelihood of left handedness among lesbians when compared to their heterosexual counterparts, lower birth weights for homosexual males when compared to their older heterosexual brothers, less asymmetric brain functioning for homosexual men and heterosexual women than for heterosexual men,[53] greater left asymmetry in finger print ridges for gay males,[54] and differences in the length ratios for index and ring fingers in homosexual and heterosexual females.[55]

In 1990, Simon LeVay may have found another significant difference in the characteristics of homosexual men. Comparing the brains of homosexual men who had died of AIDS to brains of heterosexual men and women who also had died of AIDS, LeVay found that one section of the hypothalamus (INAH3) was significantly smaller in the women under study than the heterosexual men. He also found that on average the INAH3 in homosexual males was one-half the size of those found in heterosexual males. In 2001, William Byne, Stuart Tobet, and several colleagues reported on a follow-up study examining the anterior hypothalamus at autopsy. In their examinations they found that the INAH3 region occupied less space in homosexual men than in heterosexual men.[56] Animal studies comparing rams who displayed same-sex and opposite-sex attraction found similar patterns in hypothalamic development in heterosexual and homosexual rams.[57] This is a

Among some of the more interesting characteristics that may differentiate gay men from straight men and lesbians from straight women are their responses to different body odors or pheromones. Over the past several years, researchers from both the Karolinska Institute in Stockholm and the Monell Chemical Senses Center in Philadelphia have been investigating differences in individual responses to human pheromones based on gender and sexual orientation of the person doing the smelling and of the individual generating the body odors. Hans Berklund and his team (Berglund, Lindström, and Savic 2006) have found that homosexual men and heterosexual women show a preference for male pheromones, whereas homosexual women and heterosexual men show a preference for female pheromones. When Yolanda Martins and her colleagues (Martins, Preti, Crabtree, Runyan, Vainius, and Wysocki 2005) used body odors taken directly from individuals in the study group, homosexual men were found to prefer odors of other homosexual men over any of the other groups. As might be expected, heterosexual men found these same odors to be the least appealing. Similar patterns occurred across the board, based on gender and sexual orientation (Savic, Berglund, and Lindström 2005).

Who knows—someday we might find perfumes and colognes that are marketed not only to specific genders but also to specific sexual orientations. Should this become the case, the heterosexual woman may have to choose whether she is going to wear a perfume that she might appreciate or one that her heterosexual companion finds appealing. A lesbian, on the other hand, would be able to wear a perfume that both she and her partner could enjoy.

region of the brain that may be responsible for regulating sexual attraction and is subject to prenatal hormonal impact.

Not surprisingly, critics of a biological origin of sexual orientation have pointed to the fact that in many of these studies, the characteristic differences are not absolute. For example, in LeVay's study some homosexual men had larger INAH3 regions of the hypothalamus than some of the heterosexual men. In considering this objection, we must again consider that for many of the characteristics that differentiate males from females, the variance within the group can be even more striking than the differences between the groups. As Lauren and I prove, we have tall women and short men; we also have women with little muscle mass and women with greater muscle mass. Nonetheless, on average, men are taller and have greater muscle mass than women, and it would seem that the INAH3 region for the average male heterosexual may be larger than for the average homosexual. At the same time, it is unlikely that we are going to find one physical trait that we can look at when we are trying to pick out who is gay at the next church social or the next political rally we attend. Of course there is a theory that you can tell by the shoes that they wear.

STRAIGHT TALK

Given the ram who has absolutely no desire to make time with the cute ewe but who finds her brother to be a real turn-on, given the ease with which female bonobos go back and forth between male and female suitors, and given the exploits of young bull dolphins and the myriad of other same-sex encounters throughout the wild, it seems impossible to mount a creditable argument that sex between two females or between two males is aberrant or unnatural behavior. Although we might debate whether humans who are so inclined should or should not follow their desire to mate with someone who has the same plumbing, there is no way we can label the passion as unnatural. Our scientific and public admissions about our fellow critters in the animal kingdom have pretty well shredded that label. Whether these varying expressions of same-gender attraction are a way of building community, a basis for establishing lifelong relationships, a way to experiment with sex roles, or are just a fun night out with the girls or with the boys, these behaviors must be a part of the Almighty's plan or an outcome of evolution's general unfolding.

The differences in expression across and within animal species make it highly unlikely that we will find a single purpose for same-sex behaviors. For some animals, including some humans, same-gender sexuality is best considered a phase of development (little girls or little boys playing games with each other), and for some, it's a behavior of circumstance (prisoners in jail; boys at the all-male prep school). For others, it's one set of behaviors in a wide repertoire of behaviors (bisexual adults), and for still others, it's a dominant if not exclusive lifelong pattern (gay men and lesbians). Bottlenose bull dolphins use their early boy-on-boy escapades to establish same-sex twosomes or threesomes that will work together later in life, giving them an advantage in mating with females of the species. In stark contrast, dragonflies mount other dragonflies as a way of destroying the unlucky mountee's ability to mate with damselflies,[58] elimination of the competition as opposed to the dolphins' collaboration with comrades. For some rams, same-gender mounting is an activity that occurs only when confined they are to an all-male community, whereas others find mounting and being mounted by another ram as their singular, lifetime preference. Bonobos use same-sex behaviors to avoid or resolve conflict and to build or extend community. And for the female hedgehogs and the male lion, at least at this point, it just seems like fun.

With same-sex behaviors being used for different purposes, we have to ask whether there are any commonalities in the underlying origins for these behaviors. And could there be one simple mechanism that brings about same-gender sexual orientation? Early on in my own personal quest to find an answer, I proposed what I now recognize to be a rather naïve hypothesis to a colleague who is a biogeneticist. When I offered my ideas to Matt, he looked at me politely—I was a senior university administrator, and he was a bright, but nonetheless junior faculty member—with what appeared to be pity in his eyes, handed me a book by an early mentor of his, asked me to read the relevant parts, and then sent me directly to the stacks at the library. I suspect, but can't prove, that he then closed his office door and laughed for an hour or so.

After untold days in the library turned into weeks and weeks into months, and after I'd dragged Matt and others who could help me understand into conversation after conversation, I finally emerged from a literature review worthy of at least a master's thesis, armed with a new lexicon and the answers to my questions: (a) Although we aren't sure, we have some evidence that leads us to keep looking for common origins across species, and (b) there is almost certainly no single neat little mechanism, be it biological or environmental, that serves as the sole trigger for same-gender sexual orientation. Hormones are likely at work in at least some animals, and genetics are definitely another piece of the puzzle.

Does environment contribute to same-sex activities? Most definitely when they are behaviors of circumstance (the boys of Aranda and the men in San Quentin). And environment certainly moderates the way humans express homosexual and bisexual orientations within different cultures—more openly in some than in others, for example. But the evidence that poor parenting contributes to homosexuality is highly questionable at best. Quite to the contrary, it seems more likely that homosexuality would be a trigger for negative parenting behaviors because of parental bias or discomfort. It also appears that the mechanisms that trigger homosexuality in females are, at least in part, different from those that trigger homosexuality in males. And the biological research, in the form of the twin studies and the identification of differences in secondary characteristics, suggests that contrary to the ethnographic research (e.g., Lisa Diamond's interviews with women engaged in same-sex behaviors), homosexuality in women is more strongly influenced by genetics than it is among men. What makes Joan homosexual is probably different from what makes John homosexual.

It's worth mentioning that even those who oppose acceptance of homosexual behaviors in humans have taken note of the strength of the evidence supporting a biological link. Alan Medinger, in writing on conversion or reparative therapy, suggests that there are some boys who may have a biological predisposition to gender nonconforming behavior, and radio evangelist Albert Mohler talks about the day when mothers and fathers will be able to select prenatal therapy to eliminate homosexuality in their unborn children.[59]

Is lifelong homosexuality biological? Yes, at least in part. How much of the biology is genetics and how much is hormonal is still to be determined, but there is definitely a genetic component, and most likely, both play a role. Did lack of attention from my father cause me to be gay? Quite frankly, hell no! Was it my father's or mother's genes? I don't know for sure, but there's some evidence that would support either possibility.

AND NOW, BACK TO OUR MOVIE

So how does our adventure flick end? How does this sound—Laura Croft and Robert Langdon are piecing together several of the pages they discovered and are deciphering the text, while Brother Egad is listening in through an open window. Horrified by what he hears, Egad runs off to tell the Abbot Josephus the conclusion he has drawn from the deciphered text: "Master, Langdon and Croft have finally found the origin. God save us, it is nature; our orientation is controlled by genetics." When Josephus hears these words, he understands what God wants him to do. He must release these findings, with his own interpretation imprinted on the information: "Now that we know the cause of the disease, God-fearing people must find the cure." There will be no liberty from this discovery; there will only be a new battle.

As the abbot begins preparing his plans, the camera pans back to our adventurers, who are in the midst of working on a last piece of text that they can't quite decipher, that is until Laura turns the paper over and, reading upside down, translates the last line: "Thus ends the first step in the journey of man's love for man and woman's love for woman." And yes, just as you expected, the page is torn after that inscription. Voila, we have our sequel—The Book of Origins: Finding Chapter 2, the Second Step.

NOTES

1. Bieber et al. 1962
2. Hamer, Hu, Magnuson, Hu, and Pattatucci 1993.

3. Rice, Anderson, Risch, and Ebers 1999.

4. It should be noted that there remains a continuing hesitancy to explore these occurrences of same-sex behaviors on the part of some researchers, who are unable to find funding or fear being labeled or marginalized as a result of their research (Sommer and Vasey, 2006).

5. Watanabe and Smuts 1989.

6. Bagemihl 1999; Sommer and Vasey 2006.

7. Bagemihl 1999; Sommer and Vasey 2006.

8. Bagemihl 1999.

9. Hendrickson 2005; Kurdek 2004.

10. Bagemihl 1999.

11. Bagemihl 1999; Mann 2006.

12. Kotrschal, Hemetsberger, and Weib 2006.

13. Bagemihl 1999.

14. Goldstein 2003; Larsson and Svedin 2002.

15. Crompton 2003.

16. Bagemihl 1999.

17. TFP Committee on American Issues 2004.

18. Furth and Hoffman 2006 in Sommer and Vasey, 294–316.

19. J. Massey 2006 in Sommer and Vasey 107–130.

20. Vasey 2006 in Sommer and Vasey 173–204 .

21. Ibid.

22. Bagemihl 1999.

23. Bartos and Holeckova 2006; Furth and Hoffman 2006; Yamagiwa 2006.

24. Irving Bieber as cited in National Association for Research & Therapy of Homosexuality 2004.

25. Henry 1948.

26. Moberly 1983; Nicolosi 2006.

27. Bieber et al. 1962; Medinger 2000; Nicolosi 2006.

28. Floyd, Sargent, and DiCorcia 2004; Friedman and Downey 2007.

29. N. Sullivan 2003.

30. Schwartz 1998.

31. Halperin 1989.

32. Boswell 1989; Holland 2004; Hubbard 2003.

33. Herdt and Stoller 1989.

34. Parker 2007.

35. Pinckard, Stellflug, Resko, Roselli, and Stormshak 2000.

36. Bailey, Pillard, Neale, and Agyei 1993.

37. Bailey and Pillard 1991.

38. Kirk, Bailey, Dunne, and Martin 2000.

39. Kendler, Thornton, Gilman, and Kessler 2000.

40. Hall and Kimura 1994; Sommer, Ramsey, Mandl, and Kahn 2002; Powledge 1993; Turner 1994.

41. Bruder et al. 2008; Gliding, Bolton, Vincent, Melmer, and Rutter 1997.

42. Edwards, Dent, and Kahn 1966.

43. Mustanski, Chivers, and Bailey 2002; LeVay 1996.

44. Hamer, Hu, Magnuson, Hu, and Pattatucci 1993.

45. Hu, Pattatucci, Patterson, Li, Fulker, Cherny, Kruglyak, and Hamer 1995.

46. Mustanski, DuPree, Nievergelt, Bocklandt, Schork, and Hamer 2005.

47. Pinckard, Stellflug, Resko, Roselli, and Stormshak 2000.

48. Mustanski, Chivers, and Bailey 2002.

49. Ibid.

50. Blanchard 2004.

51. Op cit, 13–14.

52. Hall and Schaeff 2008; Roselli, Resko, and Stormshak 2002; Small 1995.

53. Hall and Schaeff 2008; Mustanski, Chivers, Bailey, and Kirk 2000.

54. Hall and Kimura 1994.

55. Hall and Love 2003.

56. Byne, Tobet, Mattiace, Lasco, Kemether, Edgar, Morgello, Buchsbaum, and Jones 2001.

57. Roselli, Larkin, Schrunk, and Stormshak 2004; Pinckard, Stellflug, Resko, Roselli, and Stormshak 2000.

58. Dunkle 1991.

59. Medinger 2000, 48; Mohler 2007.

4

Sacred Scriptures and Homosexuality

A number of years ago, I was sitting in my office at the university when our secretary buzzed me to tell me that a Reverend Hayas was on the phone and to ask if I could take the call. Don Hayas was the minister at the church my mother attended, the church where I was baptized and confirmed and where I served as an altar boy. My first thought was, what terrible thing has happened in the family, and why wasn't one of my sisters calling me?

When Gerri connected Don and me, he apologized if the call had startled me—which of course it had—but he was wondering if I was coming back to Cleveland for my eldest niece's wedding and if I planned on attending church on the Sunday after the wedding. If so, Don hoped we could have a conversation on the Friday or Saturday of the wedding before the Sunday service. As he said these words, I immediately understood where the conversation was going. There would be no Holy Eucharist at the wedding—Lutherans aren't as liturgical as Catholics or Episcopalians—but there would be communion at the Sunday service, and Don wasn't sure if I could receive it. Evidently, he had recently heard that I was gay and felt he couldn't in all good conscience serve me the body and blood of Christ unless I repented of this sin. How he hadn't known I was gay before this is beyond me, but that's another story.

As my blood pressure began to rise, I suggested to Don that I would prefer to talk before arriving in Cleveland but was on my way to a meeting; I asked if I could call him later that week, so that we could have the conversation over the phone. He said yes, and we scheduled a time for what would be the first of two different conversations on the topic—one on the phone and one in person.

That afternoon there were calls to my siblings to tell them what had happened; my brother Stan, a federal prosecutor in Texas, suggested I wait to talk to Don until Stan got to Cleveland, and we could go together. Although Stan and I see the world from very different political perspectives, even today he remains my older and on occasion protective brother. There was also a call to Frankie White, the minister of the Metropolitan Community Church in Jacksonville and someone I would occasionally run into in the community. Frankie suggested that I might look in our university library to see if we had a copy of John Boswell's text *Christianity, Social Tolerance, and Homosexuality.* She assured me that anything I might want to know about biblical passages that may or may not have talked about homosexuality was covered in this book.

That night, as I sat in bed reading Boswell's text, I couldn't put it down. For the first time in my life, I was reading a scholarly and detailed accounting of the biblical passages that were so often used to denounce gays and lesbians. It was an accounting that introduced me to a whole new—new for me, that is—way of understanding the story of Sodom and Gomorrah, the Holiness Code in Leviticus and Paul's passages. The understanding of the Sodom and Gomorrah passage that Boswell offered was the same one that Jesus pointed to in Matthew 10.

Why hadn't I been exposed to these different interpretations of the Bible earlier in my life? I spent a lot of time as a catechumen learning the differences between transubstantiation, consubstantiation, and transignification (the different ways Christians view communion or the Eucharist) and the different biblical passages that supported infant versus adult baptism, but no one told me or even hinted that there might be multiple ways to read these passages that had been used to assign me to the margins of society. I had taken a course on the Old Testament as an undergraduate from a professor who had worked with the Dead Sea Scrolls, and I do remember talking about the Holiness Codes in Leviticus and Sodom and Gomorrah, but our class discussions didn't even touch on homosexuality. That was a topic that remained hidden in the curriculum then, as it often does today.

As I read and studied Boswell, I felt a flood of emotions. At first, I felt armed and ready to do battle with Don. Bring on the arguments; I was ready to handle each and every one. At the same time, I felt sadness and anger about the roadblocks that had kept me from going to the seminary, roadblocks that didn't have to be there. And then later, after some struggle, came a sense of calm and peace within myself, a calm that comes with understanding. Along with this peace and calm came a sense of curiosity about all of the other things I didn't know about myself as a gay man.

Of course, for Don and those who believe as he does, opposition to homosexuality is firmly rooted in these same passages and the various religious dogmas that have arisen from them—beliefs that would be threatened by acknowledging the rights of homosexual and bisexual individuals. For Don, homosexual behavior was a clear sign of a godless and failing society. And in voicing his opposition, as expected, he pointed to these passages as the basis for his convictions.

Responding to these perceived affronts to religious laws, many who hold conservative faiths are prepared to prosecute same-sex behaviors to the fullest extent possible within the prevailing standards of the body politic. In Islamic theocracies such prosecution may range from prison terms to capital punishment. In Western cultures this translates into more subtle and tactical efforts to limit what have been labeled as special rights: nondiscrimination in the workplace, the legal right to adopt the children of life partners, domestic partner benefits, and so forth. In pursuing the conservative agenda, some have also begun to assert that it is conservatives who are the oppressed group, claiming that with the onset of gay rights, those who hold conservative beliefs are losing the rights to freedom of speech and religion[1] and suggesting that the only way to keep these freedoms secure is to deny liberties to the homosexual minority.[2]

WHAT ARE THESE SCRIPTURAL PROHIBITIONS?

If we are conservative Jews, Christians, or Muslims, we will often begin our arguments against homosexuality with the story of Sodom and Gomorrah as found in Genesis 18 and 19. We then reaffirm our opposition with two passages from the Holiness Codes found in Leviticus 18:22 and 20:13. If we are Muslim, the assumed prohibitions from Genesis are echoed in four verses in the Qur'an that retell the story of Sodom and Gomorrah. For many Christians among us, the Old Testament prohibitions are further supported in three of Paul's epistles: the Letter to the Romans and the First Letters to the Corinthians and to Timothy.

Others of us who are Jews, Christians, or Muslims may look at these same passages and find quite different interpretations. And if we are nonbelievers or from different faiths, we may well find these scriptures irrelevant to our lives.

Sodom and Gomorrah

If we use the Torah (Old Testament or Qur'an) as part of the rationale for opposing homosexuality, we are likely to believe that Sodom and Gomorrah were destroyed because of the sin of homosexuality. But Boswell and a number of other scholars point to a different understanding of these passages. They provide an alternative understanding of the Sodom and Gomorrah story, which is consistent with other scriptural passages. Based on these readings of Genesis, the sins that led to the destruction of these two cities are more accurately described as sins of hate and arrogance and sins of inhospitality toward the children and messengers of God—an interpretation consistent with the Gospel message and with Jesus's direct reference to Sodom and Gomorrah.

In telling the story of Sodom and Gomorrah, the author of Genesis begins with YHWH (God) and two angels appearing before Abraham. Upon their arrival, Abraham opens his house to the three visitors from heaven, setting a feast before them. As they eat, YHWH informs Abraham, now over 100 years old, that they have come to tell Abraham and his wife, Sarah, a woman of 90-plus years, that they will have a son to be named Isaac. Considering her age, Sarah laughs at the prospect of giving birth to a child. But she is assured by God that this will indeed happen.

Upon leaving his tent, Abraham, YHWH, and the angels walk toward the city of Sodom. In their conversation, YHWH reveals to Abraham that he intends to destroy Sodom and Gomorrah because of the wickedness displayed by the citizens of these cities. Abraham's nephew Lot lives in Sodom. In response to this news, Abraham begins to negotiate with God to spare the cities for the sake of the few righteous men and women who live there. YHWH finally relents and says that if the angels can find 10 such men and women, he will spare the cities.

Upon arriving in Sodom, the two angels are met by Lot. At Lot's insistence, the angels forgo their plans to spend the night in the streets of the city and take shelter in his house. In accord with his faith, by offering the protection of his house, Lot assumes responsibility for the well-being and safety of the two strangers.

As they settle in for the evening, the house is surrounded by the men of the city, who insist that Lot send the angels out: "And they [the men of Sodom] called unto Lot, and said unto him: Where are the men which came in to thee this night? Bring them out unto us, that we may know them."[3] Lot replies: "I pray you, brethren, do not so wickedly. Behold now, I have two daughters which have not known man; let me, I pray you, bring them out unto you, and do ye to them as is good in your eyes: only unto these men do nothing; for therefore came they under the shadow of my roof."[4]

Hearing this conversation between Lot and the men of the city, the angels proceed to bring Lot back into the house, blind the would-be attackers, and warn Lot to leave with his family before YHWH destroys the city. The next day, Lot and his family leave the city as God begins to destroy the two cities.

If we believe that the story of Sodom and Gomorrah addresses the issue of homosexuality, we build our case on the assumption that the word *know* (*yada*) is meant to imply that the men of the city intended to have sexual relations with the angels and that these sexual relations provide evidence of rampant homosexuality among the inhabitants of Sodom. Based on this intent, we propose that God destroyed Sodom in response to pervasive homosexuality.

If we read the passage somewhat differently, we may offer three objections to this interpretation of the Genesis passages. The first and most questionable of these objections posits that *yada* may have no sexual connotation in this text.[5] This argument is premised on the fact that the word *yada* (know) is used 942 other times in the Old Testament, and in only 10 of these cases does it imply sexual relations.[6] The argument against using this story as a condemnation of homosexuality is supported to some degree by the fact that in each of the 10 cases where *yada* is related to sex it clearly refers to heterosexual intercourse. In the remaining 932 cases, the word means "become acquainted with, look over, examine, discover, become familiar with."

When Justin Volpe, a New York City police officer, anally raped Abner Louima, a Haitian immigrant being interrogated by the police, with a broomstick handle in the precinct bathroom, no one thought of this as homosexual sex; it was a crime of rape that reflected hate and disdain for those who were different.

No one has suggested Volpe was homosexual. I would, however, suggest that although Volpe wasn't homosexual, he was a sodomite according to my definition of sodomite: someone who turns his back or abuses the stranger and the less fortunate.

Although this argument may have some merit, the rest of the passage seems to contradict the objection—specifically, the fact that *yade* is also used in reference to Lot's daughter (*I have two daughters which have not known man*), where there seems to be a clear intent of sexual misconduct.[7]

A second and more convincing argument against interpreting Genesis 19 as a condemnation of homosexuality asserts that we should not conflate the intended rape of the two unknown men with homosexuality—the mutually agreed-upon intimacy between members of the same-sex. If the intent of the men of Sodom was the rape of the angels of God, such actions are much more consistent with the interpretation that the sin of Sodom is the sin of hatred of the other and the indifference to those who are strangers. The rape of a male is far from consensual sex (homosexuality). Do we condemn heterosexuality when we condemn the gang rape of a young girl or do we condemn the violence of the act? Acts of male-on-male rape are more likely to be committed by heterosexual men in prison or men who do not identify themselves as homosexual in non-prison settings. In both cases it appears that these acts serve to humiliate, control, and demean the victim.[8]

For those of us who interpret the passage in this manner, the story of Sodom and Gomorrah is about hostility toward those who are different and an unwillingness to help those in need. In this interpretation, the command to send the angels out to the men on the street reflects the men of Sodom's distrust of foreigners, a distrust exacerbated by their earlier defeat and capture at the hands of the Assyrians[9] and by the fact that the angels are being hidden by Lot, who himself is a foreigner among the people of Sodom.

The third argument against believing that the story of Sodom and Gomorrah is a condemnation of homosexuality is based on other biblical references to Sodom and Gomorrah. Other Torah (Old Testament) passages support the interpretation that the sin of Sodom was the sin of hate and self-interest instead of caring for the poor and strangers among us: "Behold, this was the iniquity of thy sister Sodom, pride, fullness of bread, and abundance of idleness was in her and in her daughters, neither did she strengthen the hand of the poor and needy."[10] And in the words of Jesus as he is sending his disciples out, "And whosoever shall not receive you, nor hear your words, when ye depart out of that house or city, shake off the dust of your feet. Verily I say unto you, it shall be more tolerable for the land of Sodom and Gomorrah in the day of judgment, than for that city."[11]

It is not until 93 C.E., 60 years after Jesus died according to some traditions, that we find any attempt to link this chapter of Genesis to sexual behavior. In that year, the Jewish historian Flavius Josephus presented his interpretation that the men of Sodom intended to have sex with the angels. In writing *Jewish Antiquities,* he was also the first person to introduce the term sodomite linked to homosexuality: "The Sodomites, however, lusted after the handsome young men, but Lot told them to refrain their passions."[12] Prior to Josephus's interpretation, the term "sodomite" was not linked to sexual behavior.

In considering the sin of Sodom in our own lives, we might want to reflect on how we treat the other, the stranger, the poor, and the different. Lot is saved because he took in and protected the strangers, again recalling our treatment of the poor and oppressed and the immigrant.

Leviticus

If we label homosexuality as a sin, we are also likely to point to two passages in the Holiness Codes found in Leviticus chapters 17 through 26. These chapters of the Torah present rules that cover a wide range of behaviors, from worship and sacrifice to the purchase and the treatment of slaves and from the lives of priests to dietary practices and food preparation. In this registry of rules, Leviticus 18 and 20 have several passages governing sexual relationships, including "Thou shalt not lie with mankind, as with womankind: it is abomination"[13] and "If a man also lie with mankind, as he lieth with a woman, both of them have committed an abomination: they shall surely be put to death; their blood shall be upon them."[14]

These two passages seem pretty straightforward: men aren't supposed to bed down with other men. So doesn't that pretty well settle the case for the biblical prohibition on homosexuality? At first glance it would seem so, but the issue is complicated by the fact that every non-Jew and most contemporary Jews choose to ignore many of the prohibitions mentioned in the Levitical litany of thou-shall-nots, claiming that particular verses don't apply to today's society. Therefore, we have to ask ourselves why we honor these two passages but ignore so many of the other verses in the Holiness Codes.

In Greek translations of the Holiness Codes, the various rules are divided into two categories: violations of law or justice (inherently evil) and ritual or ceremonial impurities (unclean acts). In the Greek translations, both Leviticus 18:22 and Leviticus 20:13 fall into the ritual impurity category.[15] This category also includes the following passage: "And if a man shall lie with a woman having her sickness [period], and shall uncover her nakedness; he hath discovered her fountain [blood], and she hath uncovered the fountain of her blood: and both of them shall be cut off from among their people."[16]

Non-Jewish and contemporary Jewish societies have chosen to ignore many of the statements set down in the Holiness Codes. This is especially true when these passages fall into the category of ritually unclean acts, such as the following examples: "The wages of a hired man are not to remain with you all night until morning" (you have to pay your housepainter each and every day, not when the job is finished);[17] "the daughter of any priest, if she profanes herself by harlotry, she profanes her father; she shall be burned with fire" (rather a stiff penalty for a minister's daughter who is having sex before marriage);[18] "as for your male and female slaves whom you may have—you may acquire male and female slaves from the pagan nations that are around you" (biblical permission for at least some types of slavery).[19] Although almost all of us accept that most of the ritual passages don't apply to us and our society, we continue to use Leviticus 18:22 and Leviticus 20:13 in denouncing homosexuality. If we are to be honest with ourselves, we must ask how we decided which passages we will enforce and which ones are no longer part of our contemporary code. There certainly is no scriptural reason for our selection process. If we keep the passages about a man lying with another man, according to the original codes, we have to keep all of the Holiness Codes. If we aren't keeping all of the ritual (unclean) laws, why did we retain these two?

In many ways, Paul was the driving force in the spread of Christianity. He also may have been one of the most conflicted men of the early church: "I can see my body follows a different law that battles against the law that my reason dictates. This is what makes me a prisoner of that law of sin which lives inside my body. What a wretched man I am! Who will rescue me from this body doomed to death." (Romans 7:23–24, NAB). What was the sin that lived inside Paul's body? It has been suggested that Paul was himself conflicted by his own homosexuality.

Such battles between religious fervor and self-loathing would certainly not be unique to Paul. Michael Wigglesworth, a Puritan minister and chaplain at Harvard in the late 17th Century, sits as one of the many historic examples. In his 1662 poem *The Day of Doom*, Wigglesworth presents a picture of the Judgment Day and cautions Christians about the punishments that can be expected. As he wrote his public and well received poetry, Wigglesworth also kept a secret personal diary: "Such filthy lust flowing from my fond affection to my pupils, whiles in their presence . . . I confess myself an object of God's loathing as my sin is of my own and pray God make it no more to me" (Bray 1996, 157).

Epistles of Paul

In addition to the passages in Genesis and Leviticus, Christians also point to three passages found in Paul's epistles. Some Christians hold that these three passages provide clear biblical prohibitions against homosexuality. Other Christians, hold that these New Testament passages fall short of condemning homosexual behaviors, suggesting instead that we are working with mistranslations and misinterpretations of the original biblical texts.

Two of the three Pauline passages appear in 1 Corinthians 6:8–10 and 1 Timothy 1:9–10:

> Know ye not that the unrighteous shall not inherit the kingdom of God? Be not deceived: neither fornicators, nor idolaters, nor adulterers, nor effeminate [malakoi], nor abusers of themselves with mankind [arsenokoites], nor thieves, nor covetous, nor drunkards, nor revilers, nor extortioners, shall inherit the kingdom of God.[20]

> Knowing this, that the law is not made for a righteous man, but for the lawless and disobedient, for the ungodly and for sinners, for unholy and profane, for murderers of fathers and murderers of mothers, for manslayers, for whoremongers, for them that defile themselves with mankind [arsenokoites], for menstealers, for liars, for perjured persons, and if there be any other thing that is contrary to sound doctrine; according to the glorious gospel of the blessed God, which was committed to my trust.[21]

If we believe that these passages condemn same-sex behaviors we may turn to more contemporary translations of the Bible to make our point. For example, the God's Word Bible translates the two terms *malakoi* and *arsenokoites* in 1 Corinthians as a single word: homosexual. In the Darby Bible the two terms are translated as "those who make women of themselves, [those] who abuse themselves with men." And in the World English Bible the terms are translated as "male prostitutes" and "homosexuals."

For the term *arsenokoites* in 1 Timothy, the God's Word Bible again uses the term *homosexuals,* the Darby Bible uses the word *sodomites,* and World English Bible uses the term *homosexual.* In contrast, scholars who question the use of these two passages in condemning homosexuality take issue with these contemporary translations of the Greek words *malakoi* and *arsenokoites.*

As Boswell[22] points out, the literal translation of *malakoi* would be the word *soft* and is translated as such in Luke 7:25 and Matthew 11:8: "a man clothed in soft raiment." Boswell and McNeill[23] suggest that when used in a moral sense, *malakoi* is more accurately translated as given to excess, self-indulgent, or immoral or, possibly, as masturbator. In contrast, the term *arsenokoites* is more difficult to translate and does not appear elsewhere in the Bible. In Romans 13:13, Paul uses the root word *koitai* to refer to wanton or excessive behavior, but the whole word is unseen before this passage. Boswell and McNeill suggest that prior to the fourth century, this term most likely meant a male prostitute, a role filled by men who were more likely to engage in heterosexual sex. The Vulgate Bible, a fourth-century Latin translation, uses *masculi concubitors* (male concubines) for the word *arsenokoites,* a phrase that supports the definition suggested by Boswell and McNeill.[24] It is only in recent times that *arsenokoites* has been translated as homosexual and without any historic basis for this shift in translation.

If we use Boswell and McNeill's recommended translations for *malakoi* and *arsenokoites* the passages from 1 Corinthians and 1 Timothy become:

> Know ye not that the unrighteous shall not inherit the kingdom of God? Be not deceived: neither fornicators, nor idolaters, nor adulterers, nor gluttons [malakoi], nor male prostitutes [arsenokoites], nor thieves, nor covetous, nor drunkards, nor revilers, nor extortioners, shall inherit the kingdom of God.
>
> Knowing this, that the law is not made for a righteous man, but for the lawless and disobedient, for the ungodly and for sinners, for unholy and profane, for murderers of fathers and murderers of mothers, for manslayers, for whoremongers, for male prostitutes [arsenokoites], for menstealers, for liars, for perjured persons, and if there be any other thing that is contrary to sound doctrine; according to the glorious gospel of the blessed God, which was committed to my trust.

The third Pauline passage, which is the New Testament passage most often used in condemning homosexuality, is taken from the Epistle to the Romans and clearly refers to same-sex behaviors:

> For this cause God gave them up unto vile affections: for even their women did change the natural use into that which is against nature; and likewise also the men, leaving the natural use of the woman, burned in their lust one

---

One interpretation is that for same-sex behaviors to be a sin, these behaviors must be in conflict with one's own nature, and some suggest that support for this interpretation can be drawn from a highly unlikely and certainly unintended source.

> Saint John Chrysostom in his Epistolam ad Romanos (circa 390 c.e.) wrote, "Likewise, [Paul] casts asides with these words every excuse, charging that they not only had [legitimate] enjoyment and abandoned it, going after a different one, but that spurning the natural, they pursued the unnatural" (Boswell 1980, 360).

toward another; men with men working that which is unseemly, and receiving in themselves that recompence of their error which was meet.[25]

The question raised in this passage is whether the denunciation of these same-sex behaviors applies to individuals who are inherently or biologically homosexual. This question is predicated on the use of the phrases "did change the natural use" and "leaving the natural use," both implying that the individuals had abandoned an instinctive or essential inclination toward heterosexuality as they stepped away from their inherent understanding of God. For those of us who read Romans 1 from this point of reference, if a same-sex behavior is a sin, the behaviors must conflict with the rule of nature or with the nature of the individual. Examples of such occurrences might be found among prison populations. However, if the same-sex behaviors are an expression of nature and the individual's natural drives, such behaviors between committed adults can be taken as a statement of love.

No doubt, if we oppose homosexuality based on scriptures, we are likely to see this argument as rubbish and self-serving. So who is right? Well, who is right about how we view adult versus infant baptism? Who is right about whether Mary had more children after she gave birth to Jesus? Who is right about marriage and divorce? Who is right about birth control? And more importantly, who has the right to say which beliefs we will honor and which beliefs we will make illegal?

> Christian views on public prayer often ignore biblical passages such as the following:
>
> And whenever you pray, do not be like the like the hypocrites; for they love to stand and pray in the synagogues and at the street corners so that they may be seen by others. Truly I tell you, they have received their reward. But you, whenever you pray, go into your room and shut the

> door and pray to your Father who is in secret; and your Father who sees in secret will reward you. And when you pray, do not heap up empty phrases as the heathens do, they think they will be heard because of their many words. Do not be like them; for your Father knows what you need before you ask Him.
>
> —Matthew 6:5–8, NOB

Matthew and Mark: The New Law

In answering the question of whether homosexuality is a sin, some of us point to the New Testament restatement of God's law as given by Jesus: "Jesus said unto him, 'Thou shalt love the Lord thy God with all thy heart, and with all thy soul, and with all thy mind. This is the first and great commandment. And the second is like unto it, Thou shalt love thy neighbour as thyself. On these two commandments hang all the law and the prophets.'"[26] When we use this statement of the law, we stress judgment of the act based on the motivation for the act: love, lust, hate, and so on. In judging a sexual act, the focus would not be on whether the act involves same-sex or opposite-sex partners, but rather on whether the act is based on love of the other and love of God. Using this point of reference, both homosexual and heterosexual acts, even among married couples, can be judged immoral if they don't occur with love, and both can be judged moral if they do occur with love.[27]

Qur'an

According to most of today's Islamists, homosexuality is a curse born of the Western world. And according to these Muslims it is a sin that occurs only rarely in countries with majority Muslim populations. According to Islamists, because same-sex sex is banned by the Qur'an, Muslims wouldn't even think of participating in such actions. And if and when they do, they need to be severely punished.

Written six hundred years after Josephus introduced his interpretation of Sodom and Gomorrah, the Qur'an holds five passages that speak about homosexual behaviors, including multiple references to the story of Sodom and Gomorrah. As might be expected based on the time these passages were written, they reflect Josephus's post-Christ interpretation: "Lot said to his people, 'You commit such an abomination; no one in the world has done it before! You practice sex with the men, instead of the women. Indeed, you are a transgressing people.'"[28]

One of these five passages taken from the fourth chapter of the Qur'an focuses on the punishment for same-sex behaviors.

If any of your women are guilty of lewdness, take the evidence of four (reliable) witnesses from amongst you against them; and if they testify, confine them to houses until death do claim them, or Allah ordain for them some (other) way. If two men among you are guilty of lewdness, punish them both. If they repent and amend, leave them alone; for Allah is Oft-Returning, Most Merciful.[29]

In today's Iran, the unspecified punishment in this passage has become death. There are similar laws in Saudi Arabia, whereas in Kuwait and Syria the punishment has become prison sentences.[30]

Although Muslims rarely suggest alternative interpretations of these passages, scholars do point to two other passages from the Qur'an that idealize the love between adult males and young boys. In both passages, one of the rewards of heaven that men can expect is to be surrounded and served by young men of beauty. "They shall be attended by boys graced with eternal youth, who will seem like scattered pearls to the beholders.[31] And there shall wait on them young boys of their own, as fair as virgin pearls."[32] These are similar to the passages that promise that Islamic martyrs will also be waited on by beautiful female virgins.

This picture of heaven is consistent with the historic literature that tells us how in many Arabic and Persian societies, same-sex love was both accepted and recounted in the poetry of the time. This acceptance of same-sex courtship followed the patterns found in other male-dominant cultures. The relationships were typically between an older and younger male, with the older male assuming the dominant role.[33] In an effort to explain the seeming disconnect between poetry that extols and romanticizes same-sex love and numerous historic accounts of same-sex partnerships on the one hand and Qur'anic prohibitions on the other, Khaled El-Rouagher suggests that it is not same-sex love that is forbidden in the Qur'an but rather anal intercourse. Thus, Muslims of the past were free to engage in courtship and often engaged in non-anal intercourse, which would have been considered a lesser offense.

El-Rouagher's argument is intriguing but less than congruent with some of the historic evidence he himself presents in his text. One of these pieces comes from the writings of an Englishman who fell into servitude and was taken to Algiers in the mid-1600s. In his letters, Joseph Pitts writes,

> This horrible sin of sodomy is so far from being punished amongst them, that it is part of their ordinary Discourse to boast of their detestable Action of that kind. 'Tis common for Men there to fall in love with Boys as 'tis here in England to be in love with Women.[34]

In presenting the view from the Muslim perspective, El-Rouagher quotes the writings of Muhamed Al'Saffar, a Moroccan scholar who was visiting Paris in 1845–46 when he wrote, "Flirtations, romance and courtship for them [Parisians] take place only with women, for they are not inclined to boys or young men. Rather it is extremely distasteful to them."[35]

Of course, today the romanticized same-sex relationships described in poetry are often denied by contemporary Muslims.

Buddhist Texts

Although same-sex behavior was certainly well known during the time of the Buddha, his direct teachings are silent on the topic, except to the extent that he demanded celibacy for monks and nuns, forbidding them to engage in any sexual activity: "Abandoning sexual relations, he observes celibacy, living apart, refraining from the coarse practice of sexual intercourse."[36] In the Parajika this celibacy is further defined to include avoidance of any genital, anal, or oral sex, regardless of partner.

For laymen and women who practice Buddhism, there is no such prohibition. But within the Buddha's teaching there is a clear statement governing human sexuality in general:

> Abandoning sexual misconduct, he abstains from sexual misconduct; he does not have intercourse with women who are protected by their mother, father, mother and father, brother, sister, or relatives, who have a husband, who are protected by law, or with those already engaged.[37]

This, the third of five precepts, is meant to govern behavior of all Buddhists.

At times, the Dalai Lama and others have asserted that this precept speaks to homosexual behavior,[38] but this is not necessarily the understanding of all Buddhist sects, some of whom feel the precept forbids those sexual acts that are forced or that would humiliate or harm either of the two parties or their families: child molestation, rape, adultery. If the sexual act is carried out in a loving relationship and is meant to enhance and build that relationship, it would not be seen as misconduct. If the act falls short of this standard, it doesn't matter if it occurs in a homosexual or heterosexual relationship, including within marriage; it is to be seen as misconduct.[39] This interpretation of the third precept stresses measuring intentions and outcomes in lieu of defining specific acts as bad or good—not all that different from the standards Jesus used when speaking about the law to the Pharisees.

The Sacred Texts: So Many Meanings

Differences in interpretations of sacred texts are not unique to the passages we use in our conversations about homosexuality. Such differences can be found throughout our religious traditions and our understandings of how society and faith interface. The Baptist, Catholic, and Quaker each read the New Testament in very different ways: expressing quite different scripturally based beliefs on papal authority, the Lord's Supper, baptism, and war. The Orthodox, Conservative, North American Reformed, and Reconstructionist Jews each find different messages in the Torah, with major differences on the authority of the Holiness Code. And Shia and Sunni Muslims will go to war against each other over their differences, as will Catholics and Protestants.

The existence of so many splinter groups in every major religion tells us that there are multiple ways to read each of our differing sacred texts. Each of these divisions is, of course, certain that they have the true understanding of their text.

TODAY'S RELIGIONS AND HOMOSEXUALITY

Despite often-recurring condemnations of same-sex love, homosexual and bisexual men and women have a history of active involvement in the religious life of most cultures, a history that extends throughout recorded time. They have been spiritual leaders in almost all, if not all, of the religions of the world, serving as the prophets and clerics, the writers of sacred music, the creators of sacred art, and so forth. Although numerical data would be impossible to reconstruct, anecdotal reports suggest that LGB men and women may have been proportionately overrepresented in these roles when compared to their overall numbers. In the most open of societies, a different sexual orientation was even seen as an attribute that contributed to this service, whereas in other societies LGB sexual orientation was often hidden or went without comment.

> Too many people—including my mother—think it's a contradiction in terms to be a lesbian and a minister. It's still not fashionable to be a queer person of faith.
>
> —Rev. Deborah Johnson, as quoted in de la Huerta 1999, p. 126

Our understanding of homosexual and bisexual involvement in contemporary religions is not well researched, but we do know that many LGB persons find that religion and communities of faith have no relevance to their lives, as is true for many heterosexuals. Their rejection of religion is often punctuated with open expressions of disdain for communities of faith, a disdain that is a direct reaction to the hostility gays, lesbians, and bisexuals have felt emanating from contemporary religious leaders and churches. Those of us who express these views ask GLB individuals who are actively involved in religion why they would remain committed to these seemingly repressive organizations.

There are also numbers of us who are homosexual or bisexual who remain committed to religion and spirituality, choosing not to walk away from religion or faith. Instead, we seek communities of faith and spirituality that are open to sexual minorities. In some cases, this means leaving our churches, mosques, or synagogues of origin to join faiths that have focused on serving the needs of LGBT individuals, such as the Metropolitan Community Church or more mainstream denominations that have pronounced their acceptance of homosexuals, bisexuals, and transgender individuals, such as the Church of Christ or specific congregations in the Episcopal Church. As readily seen in the Anglican Communion, the openness and acceptance shown by these communities of faith have caused schisms that are reminiscent of those that Paul spoke of in the early Christian church and that have led to the continuing splintering of almost all religious hierarchies.

Others of us have chosen to maintain the connections to our religions of origin through sexual minority caucuses operating on the fringes of less-than-accepting or non-accepting mainline religions: for example, A Common Bond (Jehovah's Witnesses), Affirmation (Church of the Latter Day Saints), Al-Fatiha Foundation (Muslims), Dignity (Roman Catholic), Ortho-Gays and OrthoDykes (Orthodox Judaism), or the Evangelical Network. In many instances these caucuses are working to reform these non-accepting churches. In following these various paths, those of us who are LGB find ways to integrate our sexual orientation into our belief systems.

In contrast to each of the just-mentioned paths, there are also those LGB individuals who feel compelled to stay within their religions of origin, leading secret lives filled with guilt and self-loathing. In these cases religious beliefs are in conflict with inherent nature. This can lead to severe psychological problems.[40]

SACRED TEXTS AND PUBLIC POLICY AND DISCOURSE

The use of religious belief and scriptural texts to fight against acceptance of homosexuality calls all of us to confront the same questions we face in a number of contemporary debates. What is the rightful place of religion in setting public policy? And if sacred scripture has a place in our discussions, whose scripture and whose interpretation of that scripture do we use?

For some, the political decisions a nation makes must be synonymous with our personal religious beliefs. Those who believe this way are likely to prefer that we all lived in a modified theocracy, even when they claim that isn't their preference. At the same time they are likely to object to those theocracies that teach another point of view. We may well think, "A nation that reflects Christian faith would be idyllic, but Islamic governments are repressive."

In his 1986 *Letter to the Bishops of the Catholic Church on the Pastoral Care of Homosexual Persons*, Pope Benedict XVI (then Joseph Cardinal Ratzinger) exhorted all Catholic clergy to resist the "effort in some countries to manipulate the Church by gaining the often well-intentioned support of her pastors with a view to changing civil-statutes and laws." Challenging these efforts, Benedict admonishes, "In assessing proposed legislation, the Bishops should keep as their uppermost concern the responsibility to promote and defend family life"—not individual freedom.

I well remember the calls I received when my university accepted the gift of a bronze statue of Gandhi: "This is not the kind of art work that should be placed on a public university campus. Why are you supporting Hinduism?" Nor can I forget the calls and e-mails I get when our gay and lesbian student organization sponsors a speaker on LGBT issues: "Why are you allowing this non-Christian to speak to your students? How dare you support someone who promotes this sinful life!"

Others suggest that our political choices should reflect an overarching sense of morality that need not be perfectly congruent with any individual faith. Instead, our political decisions must leave room for each to practice her, or his, own creed, as long as this creed does not impinge on the rights of fellow citizens.

> For the first three centuries after Christ's death, Christians were persecuted by the Romans. When Emperor Constantine demanded that Christianity become the religion of the state, we saw two recurring phenomena begin: Christians persecuting non-Christians and Christians supporting non-Christ like practices that were congruent with prevailing governmental policy (McLaren 2006).

As has been true throughout much of history over the past two millennia, many of us hold that our scripture and our religious teachings should inform and even dictate social mores and national laws. This is the only way to ensure the fulfillment of our ideals and to guarantee the continuation of the society. Our nation ought not make decisions that deviate from our religious doctrines. As the center of our ethical codes, religious teachings must be the foundation of our personal choices and our national policy. When others suggest different standards for setting policy, we are likely to assert that our faith, the faith of our fathers, should guide all political and ethical decisions. We may also identify these other people as modern-day infidels or heretics.

> A clear example of one of the conflicts between religious beliefs occurred in Afghanistan in March 2006, when a Muslim was charged with abandoning Islam for the sake of his newly adopted Christian faith. Under strict reading of Islamic law, Abdul Raham was threatened with execution for his conversion. Not surprisingly, Christian groups in the United States were outraged over this conservative reading of the Qur'an and the use of this conservative reading as foundation for public policy.

These attitudes lead us into a number of conflicts that dominate much of our public debate. From an American's vantage point, the use of the Qur'an in oppressing the women in Afghanistan is intolerable, but not so from the perspective of the Taliban. From a Palestinian's view, the Orthodox Jew's use of the Old Testament covenant in asserting ownership over Jerusalem is in conflict with Arab history and Islam's claim on this city. At the same time, members of the Southern Baptist Church and those of the Metropolitan Community Church will offer differing perspectives about the role of faith and scripture in deciding policy on issues related to sexual orientation. In each of these cases, religious belief serves as the seeming bedrock of the conflicting positions we take.

In light of these differences, Sam Harris[41] asks whether our civilization can continue to withstand the all-too-real consequences of using faith to dictate public policy—the wars that we have fought, the individuals who have been tortured and enslaved because they were seen as the other, our readiness to ignore reason and science all in the name of Allah or Christ or YHWH. Hasn't Western culture committed to moving beyond the idea that scripture, as *my* church teaches it, must guide the course of government?

> If those of us who are Catholic have the one true faith, isn't it our responsibility to bring all other people into our Church? And if we are the majority of the population in a given country, shouldn't we pass laws to encourage others to follow God's will as we know it? Why would others argue about national laws that conform to papal dictates on marriage and birth control or to the public veneration of Mary?
>
> If those of us who are Muslim have the one true faith, don't we have a responsibility to bring all people to Islam? And when we are the majority of the population in our country, shouldn't we pass laws that are consistent with the Qur'an and the Islamic faith, including laws that help women understand their appropriate roles and help non-Muslims adhere to the principles of Allah? Why do Westerners become so upset by our dictates that women wear burkas? Why wouldn't we establish a law that forbids a Muslim from converting to Christianity?

As Americans consider the differing perspectives within society—a government that conforms to a single body of scripture versus a government free from religious dogma—we find that often we are reading from two different texts on U.S. history: one text for those of us who believe that the colonies were founded on a principle of accommodating multiple perspectives and the other text for those who believe America was founded on the "faith of our fathers." In *American Gospel,* John Meacham illustrates how these different histories have been written.[42] If we believe that our failure to uphold Christian values is a grave concern, we are likely to read the American history that emphasizes references to God on our coins and in our Pledge of Allegiance, as well as statements such as the following from Ben Franklin: "History will also afford frequent opportunities of showing the necessity of a public religion . . . and the excellence of the Christian religion."[43] If we believe in separation of church and state, our text is likely to focus on documents such as a 1797 treaty signed by Congress that reads, "The government of the United States is not in any sense founded on the Christian Religion,"[44] as well as Franklin's declaration of doubt about the divinity of Christ[45] and Thomas Jefferson's revised Gospel that eliminates every reference to miracles or Christ's divinity.

> Our understanding of certain scriptural readings has changed over time. In 400 C.E., the Christian Church refused epileptics the right to marry or to join the priesthood, based on Mark 9:14–29. In accord with the Church's interpretation of this passage, epilepsy was caused by possession of demons or evil spirits. The restrictions based on these interpretations continued until the 1980s.

We also find different voices among the faithful who allow for pluralism. These voices range from John Shelby Spong,[46] who calls on Christians to set aside the literal use of scriptures to justify hate and the denial of personal liberty, to more conservative voices that accept a traditional interpretation of the Bible but don't believe it is their place to impose that faith on fellow citizens. A third perspective offered by John McNeill[47] and John Boswell[48] suggests that we don't need to avoid religious belief or the scriptures in considering issues such as homosexuality, but we must remain open and accepting of alternative understandings of sacred scriptures.

For the believers and nonbelievers among us who accept that society and government must respect and honor pluralism, laws that bar employment discrimination and repeal the Don't Ask, Don't Tell policy make sense, even when these actions run contrary to our individual codes of behavior. For the believers among us who accept the idea "scripture as my church teaches it must guide the course of government," such laws seem to be the work of Satan.

Despite rapidly changing perspectives about LGB rights, the strident divergence of opinion on the use and interpretation of scripture makes us question whether we will be able to reach an accord on religious objections to sexual minorities. Clearly, an individual's religious objections must be respected. But does that mean we impose one set of beliefs on all or deny freedom to the disenfranchised or marginalized?

Although recent events suggest that society can accommodate and find some balance in such debates, our long-term history tells us that societies can be extremely resistant and slow to do so. The Puritans, having been killed and prosecuted for their anti-Catholic and anti-Church-of-England sentiments, fled England for Massachusetts. Other Protestant groups sought religious freedom in the colonies of New Jersey, Pennsylvania, and Maryland. Even while fleeing religious bigotry, these various religious sects brought with them their own intolerance—a distrust of all that was Catholic. This bias continued to resonate in the opposition to John F. Kennedy's 1960 presidential campaign and, though somewhat muted and masked by common agendas on abortion and gay rights, can still be heard on the campuses of Evangelical seminaries and universities across the United States. This intolerance has not been confined to any particular faiths or been one-sided. How many mothers in Northern Ireland have cried over the dead bodies of their children? How many Iraqi Sunnis and Shiites have been killed by the other sect? How many Jews and Muslims have given their lives in Israel, the West Bank, and Gaza?

There is no way we will come to a common religious understanding, but can we afford to mask intolerance, bigotry, and hatred as righteousness and sanctity? Regrettably, our history tells us we are willing to do just that, all in the name of YHWH, Christ, Allah, and Vishnu. The best of humans have found solutions in their personal lives, focusing on one of the common messages on which each of our various religions are founded—respecting others, friend, stranger, and foe, as we would want to be respected by them.

STRAIGHT TALK

Do the sacred scriptures prohibit love and physical intimacy between same-gender partners? If you believe the story of Sodom and Gomorrah is about the sin of homosexuality, you will probably answer that, yes, scripture does prohibit same-gender love. If you believe that Sodom and Gomorrah is a story about God's anger over people turning their back on the less fortunate and abusing strangers, you will probably say no. If you believe that this a myth retold over the ages to explain some disaster, you will probably ask why we even stop to ask this question.

If you accept that Leviticus 18:20 speaks to modern civilizations, you will see the Torah, or Bible as prohibiting same-gender intimacy. But if you read this and the passages that surround it and question why we insist on following this verse but elect to ignore the other Levitical passages that come before and follow after, you may well question the use of this prohibition.

Do sacred scriptures prohibit love and physical intimacy between same-gender partners? The meaning is in the eye of the reader.

A second question we need to ask is whether our culture has an obligation to use an assumed scriptural prohibition as the basis for our social contracts and our laws. If you don't believe in these scriptural prohibitions because you don't believe in religion, or you don't think that the scriptures are correctly interpreted or that they are to be taken literally, the answer is probably easy enough—no. Why would you base social mores or laws on prohibitions that are absent any authority?

But what if you accept that there are scriptural prohibitions against same-sex love? Does that necessarily mean that laws should follow? If abstaining from same-sex relationships is a necessary step to God, this may be a code we want to help others follow, like giving to the poor, remaining faithful to our marriage vows, and avoiding lying, but that doesn't necessarily make it a basis for law. We have a number of personal and religious values that aren't codified into law. But if you view same-gender relationships as more than a personal evil and rather a call to God's judgment on the society, you will likely see this as something that must be controlled by the force of law. If God is going to send your neighbor to hell because he lives with another man, you might want to alert your neighbor to that fact. If God is going to destroy our civilization because your neighbor lives with his male partner, you might want to write a law to try to prevent that.

EPILOGUE

My mother's minister and I did have the talk on the phone and a face-to-face meeting on the Saturday of my niece's wedding. Don was surprised to learn that I had openly talked about being gay with the minister who had led that church when I was growing up and that there had been no mention of not receiving communion. He was also surprised that it was a Lutheran minister from the church I was attending in Florida who had come to the house a few years earlier to give my life partner Jimmy, his parents, his siblings, and me communion on the Easter Sunday three weeks before Jimmy died.

While we had our discussions, Don and I remained unchanged in our views on the matter. Now I had to find a way to tell my mother that I wouldn't be taking communion with her and my three siblings. She was not going to take this news easily. By this time, my father had already died, and one of Mom's greatest joys was having her four children at the communion rail kneeling together. I decided the news would wait until after the wedding. Why put her through this before such a happy celebration of love?

Rebecca's maid of honor was her younger sister, my niece Sara, who was already married with one child born and one on the way. I was staying with Sara, Mike, her husband, and her two-year-old son, Joshua. Sarah began labor just before the wedding service began, but trooper that she is she made it through the wedding and the after-wedding pictures and only then had Mike take her to the hospital to deliver Jacob. Mike was going to be at the hospital well into the night and in the morning, and someone had to watch little Joshua. And because I was staying at their house, I was the logical candidate for Joshua duty—thus, no church in the morning. I have always thought Jacob had and continues to have great timing.

With careful planning on my part, trips to Mom never included Sunday mornings. Thus, it was a couple of years before we had the conversation. By the time we did, she had already put two and two together. She told me that she and Dad should have known I was gay when I was three years old and that what Don was doing was wrong in her eyes. Although she died hoping I would change, she understood and accepted that this was who I was. The last time I entered the church I grew up in was to deliver Mom's eulogy. When she asked me to do this for her, I think she was making certain that I would be at church with her, which, of course, I would have been no matter what.

In response to Don Hayas's call and thanks to John Boswell's incredible scholarship, I began a journey to discover what the research could tell me about who I was as a Christian, gay, American male (who has a propensity to throw Buddhist philosophy and practices into the mix, a la another of my other literary mentors, Thomas Merton). As a result of this journey, today I regularly kneel at the communion rail with Michael at my side and gratitude in my heart for having a deeper understanding of the role I play in God's creation.

NOTES

1. Kovacs 2002.
2. For further discussion, see chapter 8, on the "secret homosexual agenda."
3. Genesis 19:5, KJV.
4. Genesis 19: 7–8, KJV.
5. Boswell 1980.
6. Bailey 1995.
7. Locke 2004.
8. Groth and Burgess 1980; Kramer 1998.

9. Josephus 1988 translation by Maier.
10. Ezekiel 16:49, KJV; see also Isaiah 1:17.
11. Matthew 10:14–15, KJV.
12. Translated 1988.
13. Leviticus 18:22, KJV.
14. Leviticus 20:13, KJV.
15. Boswell 1980, p. 101.
16. Leviticus 20:18, KJV.
17. Leviticus 19:13, NASB.
18. Leviticus 21:9, NASB.
19. Leviticus 25:14, NASB.
20. 1 Corinthians 6:8–10, KJV.
21. 1 Timothy 1:9–10 KJV.
22. Boswell 1980.
23. McNeill 1993.
24. McNeill 1993, p. 53.
25. Romans 1:26–27.
26. Matthew 22:37–42, KJV.
27. For further discussion on this topic, see chapter 8 in this text.
28. Sura 7:80–81, translation by Rashad Khalifa.
29. Sura 4:15–16, translation by Abdullah Yusuf Ali.
30. Human Rights Watch 2005; International Lesbian and Gay Association 2000.
31. Sura 76:19.
32. Sura 52:24.
33. El-Rouagher 2005; Kligerman 2007.
34. El-Rouagher, 1–2.
35. El-Rouagher, 2.
36. As translated from the Pali Cannon in Bodhi 2005, 245.
37. As translated from the Pali Canon in Bodhi 2005, 159.
38. Hodel 1993.
39. Harvey 2000, 411–433.
40. See chapter 5, "Reparative Therapy and the Ex-Gay Identity."
41. Harris 2005.
42. Meacham 2006.
43. Ibid., 21.
44. Ibid., 19.
45. Ibid., 21–22.
46. Spong 2005.
47. McNeill 1993.
48. Boswell 1980.

5

Reparative Therapy and the Ex-Gay Identity

In 1998, we saw a short-lived publicity campaign for ex-gay ministries in the press and on billboards across the country. In this campaign John Paulk, a former drag queen, and his wife Anne, a self-proclaimed ex-lesbian, appeared as the poster couple showing that homosexuals could alter their sexual orientation, returning to the straight life.[1] At the time, Paulk was a member of the staff at James Dobson's Focus on the Family.

The advertisements were designed to challenge the growing acceptance of gays, lesbians, and bisexuals. The assertions behind this public relations campaign were that (a) gays and lesbians could become straight, but (b) to the degree that our society was providing a positive and receptive environment for LGB people, we were discouraging them from seeking out reparative therapy programs.[2] The message was stop supporting gay men and lesbians and get them into therapy.

Even as we were first seeing this model couple on billboards and newspaper advertisements, their story began to unravel. The first questions came in the form of innuendos focused on whether Anne Paulk had ever really been a lesbian or had merely adopted that persona to join her husband's ministry,[3] allegations that remain unanswered.[4]

Then in 2000, when John Paulk was photographed leaving a gay bar in Washington, D.C., his same-sex cruising behaviors gave clear voice to the LGB community's longstanding arguments about the lasting effectiveness of such conversions.[5] Paulk was, at the time of his second outing, the president of Exodus North America, an umbrella organization that represents

Exodus, a leading ex-gay ministry, was founded in 1976, in part through the efforts of Michael Busse and Gary Cooper. In 1979, these two young men realized that they had fallen in love with each other and began considering all the emotional and psychological damage they may have inflicted in their ex-gay ministries. They flew home to tell their wives that they were leaving them to set up housekeeping as a gay couple.

Similar stories of return to gay life abound throughout the annals of ex-gay history including Guy Charles, who founded Liberation in Jesus Christ; Roger Grindstaff of Disciples Only; Greg Reid, founder of EAGLE: Ex Active Gay Liberated Eternally; and Michael Johnston, former national chair of Coming Out of Homosexuality Day (Bensen, 2003; Erzen, 2006; Haldeman, 1994; Myers and Scanzoni, 2005).

ministries focused on conversion of homosexuals. He was not the first leader of this organization to have returned to same-sex behaviors, but his status with the Dobson organization and as a poster boy for the ex-gay movement made him one of the most visible figures to fall from grace.

BACKGROUND ON EX-GAY MINISTRIES

The national and international movement that John and Anne Paulk were chosen to represent is rooted in several small evangelical ex-gay ministries that began appearing in the early 1970s. Not coincidentally, these ministries started at the same time that the American Psychiatric Association and American Psychological Association[6] voted to remove homosexuality as a category of mental illness and began to caution their members against engaging patients in conversion therapies. In response to these changes in the mental health field and to the growing militancy among gays and lesbians, highlighted by the 1969 Stonewall riots, ministries such as Love in Action (LIA) and EXIT (EX-Gay Intervention Team) began to appear in various parts of the United States. If the mainstream mental health community was disavowing the use of therapy for well adjusted lesbians and gay men, these organizations would pick up the banner, offering faith-centered programs where homosexuals could reclaim their supposedly innate heterosexual identities.

In most cases, these ex-gay ministries were founded by homosexual men and, on rarer occasions, homosexual women who felt disconnected from gay

Although most of the ex-gay ministries are based in evangelical Christian teachings, there are comparable programs in the Catholic and Jewish faiths. Courage (2000a, 2000b) is a national organization for Catholics, and JONAH: Jews Offering New Alternatives for Homosexuals (2001) is the national group working with Jews.

America. These men and women also felt rejected by and estranged from the churches in which they were raised and were working to find paths back to their foundations of faith.[7]

In the 1990s, a small group of professional mental health counselors broke ranks with the APA and joined these ministries in supporting the premise that gay, lesbian and bisexual persons could alter their sexual orientation if they so chose. Twenty years after the American Psychiatric Association voted to remove homosexuality from a listing of mental disorders, Charles Socarides, Benjamin Kaufman, and Joseph Nicolosi began an organization known as NARTH (National Association on Research and Therapy on Homosexuality). The organization provided a home for therapists who were continuing to practice conversion therapy despite the American Psychological Association, American Psychiatric Association, and American Psychoanalytic Association's concerns about the efficacy of these approaches. Each of these organizations was expressing concern about the damage that could result from these therapeutic methods.[8] These battles continue into the 21st century.

THE BASES FOR CONVERSION THERAPY

The methods that the ex-gay ministries and NARTH's members use in attempting to effect the sought-after conversions reflect hypotheses presented by writers such as Irving Bieber and Elizabeth Moberly.[9] In these theoretical models, we are told that homosexuality is a psychopathic disorder that is a reaction to poor parenting and, in particular, to the child's alienation from the same-sex parent. Boys become homosexual because their fathers distance themselves, at times in response to an overbearing mother. As the father distances himself, he fails to affirm his son's masculinity and to provide a healthy role model. With little to no support from his father, the son decides that he doesn't want to be like Dad. This, in turn, creates greater separation and even hostility between the two, often leading to the father emotionally and verbally abusing the son for being "less than a man." The separation from his father causes the son to distance himself from same-sex siblings and peers out of fear of being rejected by other males. Eventually, in an attempt to repair this loss of masculine identity, the son will sexualize the male identity and try to recapture it by sleeping with other men.

> While Freud describes homosexuality in terms not all that dissimilar from Bieber's work, Freud went on to say that to try and change homosexuality would be about as effective as to try and change heterosexuality (Bayer, 1987, p. 26).

The fact that Bieber and Moberly's theoretical models center on possible psychopathological origins of homosexuality is not surprising. In the case of Bieber's work, his theory flowed directly from earlier theories proposed by Freud. But in his model, Bieber placed emphasis on the detached father.

To confirm his theory, Bieber and nine of his colleagues carried out surveys of themselves and other psychiatric colleagues with whom they had been corresponding. In their 1962 book presenting the results of their surveys, Bieber clearly stated that he began his work with a belief that there was no biological component to sexual orientation.[10] In a detailed review of their methodology, Bieber and his colleagues also admit to having selected the survey respondents and framed the survey questions in a manner that would preclude any possible discovery of such a link.

In collecting and analyzing their data, Bieber and his research team compounded the problems of a biased design with major scientific methodological errors. The first and most damaging of these was that the responding psychiatrists reported on 106 homosexuals who were undergoing psychoanalysis, operating under a terribly erroneous assumption that the characteristics found within these patients could be generalized to a population of individuals who presented no pathology. Bieber's team failed to collect data on homosexuals who had successfully integrated their sexual orientation into their adult lives, including those who were raised in homes where parents had good marriages. If you select your sample from the people who show up in a psychiatrist's office for extensive therapy, you just can't assume that their problems are the same as John or Jane Doe who don't show up on the shrink's couch. It would be like surveying people in church and assuming that their views were representative of all people, including non-churchgoers.

Another of the several methodological errors in Bieber's study is a common one for naïve researchers—an undocumented and unproven assumption of cause-effect relationship (which came first, the chicken or the egg). Even if Bieber and his colleagues' data accurately reflected characteristics in the pathological population he studied, there is no compelling evidence that the separation between father and son was the *cause* of the son's sexual orientation. It is every bit as likely that the son's sexual orientation could have caused the separation. For example, Bob's son Terry displays some effeminate behaviors as a little boy and shows no interest in baseball, and Bob has difficulty relating to Terry's behaviors, so he pulls away from his son or begins to make fun of Terry, because Bob is uncomfortable with or disappointed in his son. Bob's separation may in turn cause Terry to feel rejected, and it is this rejection that ends up sending Terry to the psychiatrist's office. Terry didn't end up on the couch because he was gay but because his father couldn't accept that he was gay or was not masculine as Dad defined it. It wasn't the separation that caused the son to be gay; it was Dad's discomfort with the son being gay that caused the separation. Now the separation causes the son to have emotional problems. Gay sons born to fathers who can accept the differences or are unaware of the differences won't necessarily end up in the same place. (See chapter 3, on the origins of homosexuality.)

There is even greater reason for skepticism in considering Moberly's often-cited work. At the time of writing *Homosexuality: A New Christian Ethic,* which presented her theory on the origins of homosexuality and her therapeutic model for repairing homosexuality, Moberly had never treated a homosexual individual, nor had she conducted any research on the topic other than reading the works of other writers.[11] Nonetheless, it is this book that remains the most often cited source for current ex-gay ministries—a book that presents a theory void of scientific evidence.

THERAPEUTIC STRATEGIES

Over the years, different ex-gay ministries have tried various homegrown approaches in pursuing conversion therapies, including the visualization and healing prayers advocated by Leanne Payne in her Pastoral Care Ministries program and a modified form of Alcoholics Anonymous's 12-step program used by Homosexuals Anonymous.[12] In the 1970s and 1980s, some of these programs came under severe criticism for using electric shock and other forms of aversion therapy in an effort to eliminate or diminish physical arousal to same-sex stimuli.[13]

Using this method, Barry is shown a stimulus that would normally arouse him sexually—possibly a pornographic picture or a taped story of love between two men. At the same time, Barry is given an electric shock or other aversive treatment. The pairing of the stimulus and the aversive treatment is meant to diminish and eventually extinguish the romantic and sexual arousal.

One of the most extreme examples of aversion therapy or deprogramming was reported by a young woman in Cincinnati. After being abducted off the street by two young men, Stephanie Riethmiller was transported by her father and then her mother to a secluded cottage in Cedar Bluff, Alabama. For a period of seven days, she was kept hostage by three men and her mother. During the seven days, she was harassed about being a lesbian and raped by one of the men. Her mother was in the adjoining room during the rape episodes, which, her mother said, she thought were consensual (Love with an Improper Stanger, 1984).

Although a number of studies on these behavioral modification methods reported some levels of success, post-research reviews point to a number of failures and misinterpretations of the data. When clinicians followed up with the male participants treated at one center, they found very different results than originally reported. In looking at 47 participants who went through an aversive therapy program, the researchers initially reported that 12 had adapted to heterosexuality. Several years later, the researchers contacted these same 12 men. What they found was that all but two of the participants had gone back to having same-sex relationships or to using homosexual fantasies when engaging in sex with their wives. One participant couldn't be found for follow-up, and the 12th participant said he was living heterosexually but wouldn't let the researchers interview his wife.[14] In many cases, these aversive therapies also caused direct and, at times, significant harm to the person undergoing the therapy program, while failing to yield any meaningful conversions. Now Barry isn't straight, and he has additional emotional problems in relating to someone of his own sex.[15]

Today, many of the ex-gay ministry programs have adopted strategies that reflect the theories presented by Moberly. These programs are based on deterministic archetypes of the masculine and feminine: men are outer-directed, and women are inner-directed; men's brains are more specialized than are women's; men are taller, and women tend to be shorter; men have superior eye-hand coordination; men dominate, and women are subordinate; men initiate, and women respond; men have authority, whereas women have power; and men seek truth while women seek mercy.[16] Although some aspects of these archetypes are considered to be genetically inherited and immutable (e.g., height), the ex-gay ministry asserts that other assumed-to-be naturally-occurring characteristics can be abandoned in early childhood as a result of conflicts with the same-sex parent. The female homosexual child walks away from female characteristics and her mother's role model, if one is even provided. She is a child without gender identity.

In these programs men and women are asked to repair or replace their injured or missing identity. The adult homosexual must begin by bonding with same-sex peers in a nonsexual manner. In the process, she or he must begin to assume the gender characteristics that have been abandoned. Mary needs to wear makeup and high heels; Terry needs to go camping and fishing. Only after Mary and Terry have worked through this process will they be able to focus on developing loving sexual attachments with members of the opposite gender. Throughout this process, biblical teachings and faith-based communities are used to support the individual's journey back to heterosexuality.

In her ethnographic research, Erzen provided a view of how this therapy unfolds at New Hope Ministries, a residential program in San Rafael, California.[17] Up until 2007, the men at New Hope had to agree to spend a year in residence under close supervision. At first, all calls and visits from people outside the program were monitored, and the men were required to travel in groups of three, never in groups of just two, lessening the risk of sexual activity between peers while, at the same time, encouraging the men to bond with each other. In phase 2, the men could travel in groups of two, and by phase 3, they could travel on their own, within a restricted area. Only in phase 4 could they venture into nearby sinful and tempting San Francisco, and then only with someone else from the program.

As part of the ongoing supervision, the men were required to check in and out as they came and went. The videos they watched, the materials they read, and the music to which they listened had to fit within the proscribed standards that supported the mission of the program. They were not allowed to use the Internet out of fear that they might log on to pornographic sites.

While enrolled in the yearlong program, the men worked in jobs within the surrounding community. In the evenings and on weekends, they engaged in structured activities that included Bible study, prayer sessions, and mandatory church attendance at the Church of the Open Door, a nondenominational church affiliated with the ministry. Throughout the week, the men were also involved in study groups that focused on addiction studies, the nature of homosexuality as defined by the program, building a masculine identity, and opposite-sex dating. On weekends, the men would engage in overnight camping and hiking trips designed to rekindle or strengthen their male identity. At some of their sessions, the men met with heterosexual men from the community, asking these straight role models questions about the heterosexual identity.

In Erzen's text and other materials from New Hope,[18] we can see a set of recurring themes that organize this therapy program: accountability, a search for the cause of the gay identity, exposing the pain reputed to be inherent in a gay lifestyle, building a stronger relationship with Jesus, and building a new identity through personal testimony. As part of the recurring accountability theme, the men were expected to self-disclose any slips that occurred in their own behavior, as well as any infractions that they had seen others in the program make: looking at pornography, having sex, and so on. In the group activities, the men were also challenged to label the causes of their own homosexuality: recalling the poor relationships between their parents, identifying when their fathers called them "sissy," or recounting experiences of physical or sexual abuse. As they searched their pasts, the men were also expected to tell the story of their own forays into the homosexual world and the pains that these steps into homosexuality caused them: the anonymous sex, self-defined sexual addiction, the sense of emptiness, the use of drugs and alcohol, the separation from family and church. The men were taught that it was through their faith in God that they could be made new and lifted out of their pains. These revelations were to be drawn from their Bible study, their church attendance, the nurturing and close sense of community in the program, and their discussions about God's plan for them.

> The picture of gay life provided in ex-gay ministries ignores those individuals who have successfully integrated their sexual orientation into their family, work, social, and religious lives. In ex-gay ministries gay life is equated with anonymous sex, unsuccessful relationships, and separation from family and church.

During their public testimonies, the men were expected to talk about the pains of being gay, the separation from their families, confessions of their many sins, and their future in the church. Through public testimony, the men were taught to create a narrative about their lives that told the horrors of the past and set the expectations for the future, a narrative that they could rehearse and through rehearsal use as a roadmap to describe where they had been and where they were going. It was in this personal narrative that they declared their new identities.

THE MEN AND WOMEN WHO COME TO THE MINISTRIES

Those who are LGB and seek out ex-gay ministries could hardly be considered a cross-section of homosexuals in America. These ministries tend to be male-focused, with considerably less outreach to lesbians. The overwhelming majority of LGB individuals who involve themselves in these ministries are white and middle-class, from strong and conservative religious backgrounds.[19]

When they come to an ex-gay ministry, they typically do so as a result of significant conflict in their lives. Feeling guilt, they are experiencing discord in their attempts to balance family and religious lives with hidden and closeted lives as homosexuals.[20] Their sexual contacts are often anonymous and unfulfilling. With some exceptions, they have not identified themselves with openly gay or lesbian organizations and have failed to develop successful, long-term same-sex partner relationships or other social support structures. Almost all of the men and women who join these ministries report low self-esteem, and many report that they believe that they are sex addicts.

Although little data is kept on the success of these ministries, it appears that most gay men or lesbians who come to these programs leave early, disenchanted or unable to deal with the required structure. The year that Erzen spent at New Hope, 11 men joined the ministry. Seven of these 11 men left within the first two months of the program. After completing the ministry, two others returned to dating men. The two who stayed with the program reported a sense of community that allowed them to be open about their religion and their continuing struggles with homosexuality. They reported having found a place that supported them.

The men and women who go through these ministries often adopt what is referred to as an ex-gay identity. Some of them see this ex-gay identity as equivalent to being heterosexual. But more often than not, the ex-gay identity is seen as something different from a recovered innate heterosexuality. Although leaders of mainstream evangelical organizations, such as Focus on the Family, portray ex-gay conversions as transformations to heterosexuality, the men and women who lead many of the ex-gay ministries characterize this new identity in more nuanced terms:

> We are frequently asked "Do you make homosexuals into heterosexuals?" Our answer is "No, we only point the way to wholeness in Christ." . . . Do ex-gays develop an interest in the opposite sex? Yes they do. But it is just that, an interest, not a lust.[21]

> Most males [ex-gays] I have encountered continue to differ from other men in that they do not become sexually stimulated by the sight of a woman's body. . . . Most men find that a strong sexual attraction to women does not arise until they meet that one special person that comes into their life.[22]

For men who have come through the ministry, the reported conversions are even less tied to heterosexuality:

> Heterosexuality isn't the goal; giving our hearts and being obedient to God is the goal.[23] There is no such thing as a cure, you learn how to manage your life, thoughts, and desires and you achieve a sense of wholeness and a better relationship with God.[24]

> If you're coming into the program to be changed to heterosexual, you're probably going to be disappointed. If you're coming here to develop a bond with Jesus, that's what will happen, and out of that change happens.[25]

Within some ministries the goal may not even be spoken of as a conversion to heterosexuality, but rather as a goal of godly celibacy.[26]

In her work, Erzen found that ex-gay men often thought of themselves as being in flux, not gay but not heterosexual.[27] These men acknowledged that they are involved in a lifelong process that has more to do with their fight to adhere to their religious convictions than it does with their becoming straight. And for many, it is involvement in the ministry that sustains them and substitutes for intimate love relationships, heterosexual or homosexual.

EFFICACY OF REPARATIVE THERAPY

Since the inception of reparative therapy and ex-gay ministries, we have been engaged in a running battle as to how effective versus how potentially damaging such therapies might be. In considering these questions, the American Psychological Association[28] and American Psychiatric Association[29] reported that the claims of conversions have been overstated and misleading. Leaders within these and other organizations have also pointed to the paucity of sound research emanating from NARTH's clinical work.[30] In response, supporters of reparative therapy such as Fr. John Harvey have argued that although many homosexuals may not succeed in conversion, if one man or one woman does, then this proves it can happen, and reparative therapy can help others live the life of godly celibacy.[31]

In response to the often-cited lack of scientific evidence on the efficacy of reparative therapy, psychiatrist Robert Spitzer worked with advocates from ex-gay ministries and practicing members of NARTH to identify a cohort of individuals who had completed an ex-gay ministry or professional therapeutic protocol and had experienced a five-year or longer change in their sexual orientation.[32] After 16 months of repeated attempts to identify a sample that was large enough for data analyses, the organizations and therapists were able to provide Spitzer with 200 individuals from the United States and Europe that fit the criteria. Thirty-eight of these participants were themselves therapists or directors of ex-gay ministries and assumed to be highly motivated to make sure that the study proved the therapy worked.

In structured phone interviews, Spitzer asked each of these 200 participants a set of 114 closed-ended questions on topics about their pre- and post-therapy sexual orientation, attractions, and behaviors, as well as questions about the reasons for and types of therapies they pursued in seeking sexual orientation conversion. As would be expected based on the mandated selection criteria (you must have a five-year or longer change in sexual orientation), all of the participants reported significant changes in their sexual orientation and behaviors as a result of therapy. But only 11 percent of the men and 37 percent of the women reported being exclusively or nearly exclusively heterosexual post-therapy. Over 50 percent of men reported having some level of ongoing sexual attraction to males. For women, this figure dropped to 16 percent. Ninety-nine percent of the men and 100 percent of the women reported having had no same-gender sexual encounters anytime during the year prior to the survey.

The study that was intended to provide the ultimate proof of the efficacy of conversion or reparative therapies left us with significant questions about the supporting arguments and the validity of the results—the first of which has to do with success rates. With more than 1,000 therapists in NARTH and 100 or more ex-gay ministries affiliated with Exodus International, Spitzer himself questioned why it took 16 months to find 200 individuals on two continents who fit the criteria of having a change in sexual orientation that lasted for five or more years. A second question we have to ask is about Spitzer's interpretation of how significant these conversions were. Reflecting on the data reported—less than half reported memories of being exclusively homosexual before therapy—could the majority of the men and women included in this study be most accurately described as bisexual before therapy and living in the heterosexual portion of this identity post-therapy?

As shown in Spitzer's study, saying I am heterosexual to someone on the phone may not be the best proof of heterosexual versus homosexual desire. Adams, Wright, and Lohr (1996) point to the fact there are methods of measuring the degree of sexual arousal when shown pictures that have proven to yield different results than self-report surveys. In their study these researchers found that some men who claimed to be heterosexual and hostile toward homosexuals on paper pencil surveys showed measureable and significant arousal when asked to look at pictures of naked men.

The other and more persistent questions many of us have asked concern the strength of the research, focused on the accuracy of the reported results.[33] Spitzer acknowledged but dismissed these questions without answering them.[34] Could the participants remember exact details about their sexual behaviors and orientation from 12 years earlier, as required by the pre-therapy measures? Were the respondents credible, or were they biased in their responses? In developing their self-narratives, had some or all of these individuals altered or embellished their stories and by repeatedly telling their stories accepted the changes in the new narratives? Would more objective measures of sexual arousal yield different results than self-reported assessments?

Much of the other research on reparative therapy follows similar patterns. The numbers of men and women who show up seeking therapy are extremely small when compared to the numbers of homosexuals in the population. Those who do show up tend to be people who are conflicted by religious questions. When we look at the percentage of people who complete the therapy, the numbers once again shrink because many leave before the program is over. Of those who complete the therapy, about 20 percent report significant change, about half report some change, and then the remaining participants report some improvement or no change.[35] What is lacking in all of these studies is hard evidence that these few conversions are real and last over time.[36]

Although Spitzer's and others' results are highly questionable, it's important to note that some of the published research from the other side is not much better. In a survey of 202 individuals who participated in conversion therapies that averaged 26 months in length, 87 percent of the respondents reported no benefit.[37] Of the 26 ex-gays who reported some benefit, 18 also reported having slips in their behavior. Seven of the eight men who reported no slips in behavior were serving as ex-gay counselors at the time of the survey. But we need to recognize that these respondents were found by placing ads in gay publications. This not a likely source for finding men and women who might have succeeded in reparative therapy.

> In 1998, the American Psychiatric Association adopted the following position statement on reparative or conversion therapies:
>
> The potential risks of reparative therapy are great, including depression, anxiety and self-destructive behavior, since therapist alignment with societal prejudices against homosexuality may reinforce self-hatred already experienced by the patient. Many patients who have undergone reparative therapy relate that they were inaccurately told that homosexuals are lonely, unhappy individuals who never achieve acceptance or satisfaction.

While some individuals reported benefit from their therapy, some also reported some level of harm as result of the therapy. The types of harm described by the participants included lowered self-esteem, depression, and attempted suicides. But just as Spitzer didn't follow up to determine objectively how successful his reported conversions really were, these researchers did not follow up to determine how real the damage was.

Although the findings from this second study are suspect, there are other credible follow-up studies focused on aversion therapies that point to the same conclusions about the dangers of aversion therapy.[38]

In his closing discussion, Spitzer dismissed questions about possible harm from such therapy by stating that none of his participants reported any. This of course leaves unanswered the questions of harm done to the untold numbers who were not successful in therapy and those who chose not to participate in Spitzer's study.

Considering the size of the gay, lesbian, and bisexual population, it should be noted that very few members of the LGB community show up for therapy, more than half who do show up leave before therapy is completed, and only 20 percent or so of those who start complete therapy.

ETHICAL DILEMMAS

In considering the efficacy of reparative and other conversion programs, several authors have raised issues of professional ethics. Among these are questions about who is qualified to offer such programs and whether programs run by individuals who do not have any mental health counseling backgrounds should be allowed, as occurs in most ex-gay ministries.[39] According to the objections, when offered through ex-gay ministries, these programs are unregulated by professional codes of ethics, and the individuals offering therapy are often ill equipped to see the warning signs of, or to handle, significant mental health issues.

We see different sets of ethical questions arise when these programs are offered through professional therapists. The most common has to do with whether the theories proposed by these professionals constitute an attempt at remedicalizing a natural variant of human sexuality.[40] Reparative therapy is offered as a cure for homosexuality, but if it is not a disorder, why would we cure it?

An equally interesting and related ethical issue deals with the professional therapist's ability to accept and work with the individual patient's commitment to her or his religious faith. Haldeman noted that religious orientation may be an extremely compelling force in our lives and must be respected.[41] In cases where there is conflict between religion and sexuality, Haldeman asserts that the therapist should be able and willing to work with the client to discover the best course of action for that individual as opposed to prescribing a single approach for each and every person who walks into the office. The therapist must work with the client in an open and honest manner, with full disclosure about what success means (celibate homosexual versus ex-gay versus fully heterosexual) and what the success rates are.

In presenting his argument for setting different goals for therapy, Haldeman offers three different cases as examples of how this individuation might work. In one case, the client leaves therapy understanding that although he was and would remain homosexual, he could elect to remain celibate in keeping true to his religious beliefs. In the second case, the client finds a mainstream faith community that allows him to express his homosexuality in a manner consistent with his Christian beliefs. In the third case, the client discovers that as a bisexual he is most content to live in a committed heterosexual relationship, without denying or feeling guilty about his same-sex attractions. In each of these cases, the client's needs are what direct the course of therapy, not the therapist's bias. To assume that all clients need to change their sexual orientation violates principles of therapy, as would the assumption that all clients need to change their religious beliefs. It would also be a violation of therapeutic ethics to mislead clients into believing that sexual orientation can be changed by therapy without better evidence than exists today.

Sixteen-year-old Zachary Stark was forced by his parents to attend an ex-gay residential program in Tennessee. In his blog Zach discussed the damage that resulted from his forced incarceration. "[My parents] tell me that there is something psychologically wrong with me . . . I am a big screw-up to them, who isn't on the path God wants me to be on. So I'm sitting here in tears . . . and I can't help it" (Cianciotto and Cahill 2006, 1).

A fourth set of ethical dilemmas occurs when the calls for therapeutic intercessions are focused on minors.[42] James Dobson of Focus on the Family and Joseph Nicolosi of NARTH have both advocated for families to be aware of "prehomosexuality" and to work with preadolescent children in trying to prevent these tendencies. In his writings, Nicolosi spoke about his own work with a five-year-old "prehomosexual." What seems ironic and troubling about these proposals is that with homosexual children, such interventions from well-meaning parents may in fact heighten the children's feelings of separation, causing them to have even more pathologies than do the men and women who currently present themselves for reparative therapy as adults. Such pathologies can result from guilt and emotional trauma in the life of the child. Instead of being cured of homosexuality, children who go through these therapies are likely to experience diminished self-concepts caused by their failure to live up to their parents' and therapists' expectations.

THE POLITICS OF REPARATIVE THERAPY

It should come as no surprise to any of us that our professional and political agendas become blurred in discussions about the ethics and efficacy of reparative therapy. In the hopes of winning the public relations battle on the gay debates, NARTH has joined with voices from the evangelical movement to advertise reparative therapy as the alternative to homosexuality: If the poster couple can change their sexual orientations, shouldn't we expect all people to do the same? Leaders from NARTH have also adopted the strategy of accusing individuals from mainstream professional associations of unfairly attempting to silence NARTH by trying to place limits on its members.[43] In countering these accusations, professional organizations such as the American Psychiatric Association, the American Psychoanalytic Association, and the American Psychological Association[44] have accused NARTH and its leaders of misrepresenting the organizations' various official positions.

During these political battles, solid research documenting the efficacy of reparative therapy has been blatantly absent. The professionals and ministries involved have systematically failed to collect data documenting the numbers of people who have come into the programs, how long these people have stayed, and how each feels upon exit. And as highlighted by the issues in Spitzer's data collection, meaningful long-term follow-up is for all practical purposes nonexistent. Unfortunately, the science that questions conversion therapy is not much stronger, with the exception of what we can glean from Tanya Erzen's compelling ethnographic study and the data that challenges the use of aversion therapies. Throughout all of this, professionals on both sides of the aisle continue to rail against each other, with what seem to be the loudest voices supporting reparative therapy and what appear to be the largest number of voices opposing it.

In *Straight to Jesus,* Erzen[45] pointed out that during these political maneuvers, the men and women who are struggling with reparative therapy remain unheard. Feeling separated from and unwelcome in churches where heterosexuality is the rule, and unwilling to join in the battles for or against their gay-affirming brothers and sisters, the LGB men and women who are involved in reparative therapy remain frustrated by the inability to reach the promised land.

STRAIGHT TALK

If we surveyed psychologists and psychiatrists across America as to whether reparative therapy works, most professionals' answers would range from "most likely not" to "hell no!" If we narrowed our focus, asking only those mental health professionals who align themselves with NARTH the same question, we would get "yes, of course." Although the "most likely not" and "hell no!" crowd might not sound as energized as the "yes, of course" voices, it's important to keep in mind that members of NARTH are the therapists and counselors who walked away from mainstream professionals organizations because of their individual belief in the ability to cure homosexuality. Ignoring the numerous cautions expressed by the American Psychiatric and Psychological Associations, these men and women choose to engage in therapeutic practices that are founded in large part on Bieber's research, which is riddled with errors, and on Moberly's work, which is little more than supposition and speculation. And then when challenged to prove the efficacy of their work, these professionals have been unable to identify an adequate sample of successful conversions to convince any reasonable panel of scientific judges.

But what about Fr. Harvey's question: if one person becomes heterosexual, doesn't that prove that reparative therapy works? That question opens a number of other questions that pose a fairly rigid test for proving conversion. Was the person bisexual or exclusively homosexual before the therapy? Have we measured the man or woman's arousal when shown same-sex stimuli? Have we measured her or his arousal when shown opposite-sex stimuli? How long has the conversion been in place? What does the person's opposite-sex spouse say to her or his closest confidants? Just checking the box on a survey may not mean much, especially when checking the box is a sign of being normal or acceptable. And how often can or do we get these results?

My friend Peter has been married to his wife Karen for 32 years. They have four wonderful daughters, two of whom Peter has walked down the aisle. Each time Peter has stepped out on his marriage vows, it has been with a man. There have been years when he hasn't broken his vow, and then there have been years when he has broken it at least once a month. If you asked Peter's wife if he is straight, Karen would probably say yes, unless you are the closest of friends, and then she might say, "Sometimes, I am not sure." If you ask Peter, his answer would also depend on to whom he is talking and where he is in his life at that time. When Peter and I first met, he wanted to leave his wife and find the man of his dreams—he was gay and living a lie. Later he was bisexual, but unfulfilled. All through this time, if you were Peter's family, one of his clients, or his priest, Peter would tell you he is straight as an arrow. Peter never looks at heterosexual porn but loves gay porn. Is Peter gay or bisexual? I'm not sure, but he isn't straight even if he would check that on a survey as he has told me he would.

In describing the outcomes of reparative therapy, Erzen presents us with a picture of most would-be converts walking away from therapy early on. Those men who stick it out do find a level of success in the program—success that comes in the form of an ex-gay persona. In adopting this new identity, the individual separates him or herself from a gay or lesbian identity and stops engaging in homosexual activity but fails to become truly heterosexual. His or her fantasies and desires don't become focused on the opposite gender, but he or she ceases to act on his or her homosexual desires.

The road to this ex-gay identity often starts with significant conflicts between the individual's religious identity and the person's sexual orientation. It is a road littered with disappointments and struggles with family and friends. In following this particular path, the individual is promised renewed community within the church and a new identity as a heterosexual. But the new identity he or she finds is as an ex-gay, not as a born-again heterosexual, and more often than not, the renewed community is limited to joining with other ex-gays. The many who leave early say the road is too difficult; for those who stay the course, the road takes them someplace different from where they had planned on going.

In his work, Haldeman offers honest alternatives for the homosexual who holds a firm religious faith—but only after she has an opportunity to understand the different paths. No matter which path the gay man or lesbian follows, he or she is taught to be honest about and accepting of his or her sexual orientation. The end result may be a life of celibacy but not denial, or it may be a change in the person's understanding of her relationship to God. It does not demand that the individual give up either her sexual orientation or her commitment to leading a religious life. Both can coexist, if acknowledged honestly and openly.

A PERSONAL REFLECTION

Having lived an intentional year of celibacy, I can appreciate how fulfilling this type of experience can be, no matter what your sexual orientation. But it should not serve as a place to hide your sexual orientation; it ought to be a place to recognize and appreciate who you are. If you hide from yourself, the celibacy is a meaningless exercise filled with lies instead of a path to truth.

Having been in two intimate relationships with women lasting more than six months—one filled with lies about my sexual orientation and one filled with caring, fidelity, and complete honesty—I know that neither made me heterosexual. I am certainly capable of having sexual relationships with women, but that is far from being straight, and in my case, I don't even think I would be fairly classified as truly bisexual. Having opposite-gender sex or being celibate does not make a homosexual into a heterosexual. If you engage in these behaviors with an honest acceptance and acknowledgment of who you are, both behaviors can be affirming. If you enter into either of these with denial or lies, you damage yourself and those whose lives you touch.

NOTES

1. Leland and Miller 1998.
2. Haldeman 1999.
3. Carlson 1998.
4. Bensen 2003, 33–34.
5. Bensen 2003; Evangelical Press 2002.
6. American Psychiatric Association 2000; American Psychological Association 2006.
7. Erzen 2006.
8. American Psychological Association 2006; Bensen 2003; Lynch 2006; Nicolosi 2002.
9. Bieber et al. 1962; Moberly 1983.
10. Bieber et al. 20.
11. Erzen 2006; Ford 2000.
12. Erzen 2006.
13. American Psychological Association 2006; Haldeman 1994, 1999.
14. Green 1988, 564–65.
15. American Psychological Association 2006; Haldeman 1994, 1999.
16. Medinger 2000, 77–79, 84–88.
17. Erzen 2006.
18. Worthen 1995.

19. Erzen 2006; Morrow and Beckstead 2004; Spitzer 2003.

20. Erzen 2006; Haldeman 1994, 2004.

21. Worthen 1995, 151.

22. Medinger 2000, 204–5.

23. Curtis as quoted in Erzen 2006, 3.

24. Erzen, 68.

25. Hank as quoted in Erzen, 71.

26. Courage 2000a; Harvey 1996, 115–22.

27. Erzen 2006.

28. American Psychological Association 2006.

29. American Psychiatric Association 2000.

30. Cianciotto and Cahill 2006; Haldeman 1999; Morrow and Beckstead 2004.

31. Harvey 1996, 69–114.

32. Spitzer 2003.

33. Bancroft 2003; Carlson 2003; Cohen 2003; Drescher 2003; Friedman 2003; Hartmann 2003; Herek 2003.

34. Spitzer 2003.

35. Pattison and Pattison 1980; van den Aardweg 1986..

36. Green 1988.

37. Shildo and Schroder 2002.

38. Green 1988.

39. Haldeman 1999; Shildo and Schroeder 2002.

40. Bensen 2003; Conrad and Angell 2004; Morrow and Beckstead 2004.

41. Haldeman 2004.

42. Cianciotto and Cahill 2006.

43. Nicolosi 2002.

44. American Psychological Association 2006; Lynch 2006.

45. Erzen 2006.

6

The Downfall of Society

Most of us have at one time or another heard a recounting of history that tells us that societies that accepted or normalized homosexuality incurred the wrath of God.[1] In these retellings of history, same-sex behaviors are depicted as an indicator of an overall moral decay that inevitably leads to the collapse of civilizations that accept or celebrate homosexuality and bisexuality.

In their narratives, the storytellers who offer us these histories rarely if ever speak of the universality of same-sex behaviors throughout history or of the positive and significant contributions lesbians, bisexuals, and gay men have made to societies throughout time. Instead, they would ask us to limit our understanding of same-sex behaviors and LGB people to incomplete and inaccurate accounts of the Roman Empire and classic Greek civilizations, compounded by erroneous conclusions about a link between these behaviors and a degeneration of social order.

> We will tell you that 20,000 years of evolution, of societal evolution, has taught us the same thing: that a society that embraces homosexuality is a society that will not last much longer. Anybody who's studied history knows that.
>
> —Michael Savage, November 16, 2006

Their job in convincing us that homosexuality is a curse on society is made easier by the absence of information about same-sex behaviors found in most history texts and the fact that most Western biographers have not considered or have been afraid to speak about the same-sex attraction exhibited by many notable historic figures. After all, if our biologists could ignore and misinterpret the ever-present evidence of same-sex behaviors in nonhumans, it seems reasonable to expect that the historians among us would be even more inclined to use social mores as filters in writing their critical analyses: we can talk about the Da Vinci's genius but we remain silent on his sexual orientation.

These biases notwithstanding, over the past several decades, contemporary researchers have begun to challenge this longstanding record of silence and misinformation, piecing together data that suggest that same-sex behaviors have existed throughout history and across all cultures.[2] Their research also illustrates that homosexual behavior and LGB individuals are in no way associated with the decline in civilizations. Quite to the contrary, the contributions of these men and women have helped weave the fabric of great accomplishment in cultures throughout time.

In fact, evidence tells us that same-sex behaviors in proto-humans date as far back as 5 million years ago, during the late Miocene and early Pliocene eras.[3] Some researchers have uncovered prehistoric cave paintings, circa 17,000 B.C.E., that show male figures with erections engaging in what appears to be same-sex behaviors.[4] Others have found historic records that indicate that same-sex behaviors have been practiced in one form or another across most, and probably all, cultures, including the indigenous peoples of Africa, Australia, the South Pacific Islands, and North and South America.[5] And these behaviors can be found during each of the various cycles within these civilizations.[6] Of course, considering how same-sex behaviors permeate the animal kingdom, it's not surprising that we would find all of this to be true.

Regrettably, but as is almost always the case in writing history, our ancestors failed to record many elements that would have helped complete the picture. In other instances, the data that were there have been destroyed over time. And in at least some instances, those elements that do exist have been misrepresented as a result of bias or prejudice. Despite these missing and misinterpreted elements, scholars have been able to provide us with a colorful and at times tragic mosaic detailing both expressions of and societal attitudes toward same-sex behaviors—a mosaic that details societies that honor same-sex relationships at what might be considered their cultural zenith contrasted against pictures of reputed homosexual men and women being burned at the stake or committed to concentration camps and used in horrendous medical experiments.

In looking at this mosaic, we can see several patterns commonly found in other historic and biographic annals. The stories of same-sex attraction are much more detailed in portraying the lives of men than of women and in chronicling the lives of the intellectual, social, or political elite than the ordinary citizen. As with most of our histories, it isn't until more recent times that scholars began to pay close attention to the common men or women, be they hetero or homosexual. The stories of same-sex attraction also provide more examples of what we might, at least on the surface, label as bisexual behavior as opposed to exclusively homosexual. Many of the men about whom historians were writing would often, albeit not always, find it convenient to marry and have children while leading separate, but not necessarily completely hidden, lives with their male companions.

In examining the unfolding picture of cross-cultural expressions and attitudes toward same-sex behaviors, we find that the data shine as much light on the cultures in which the women and men lived as they shine on the individuals themselves. Expressions of same-sex behaviors often mimic the norms found in concurrent social conventions. This becomes apparent when we compare the age differentials between the younger and older males who often joined together in the Roman Empire and classic Greece and the age differentials for opposite-sex marriages in these same societies — teenage wives and 30-year-old husbands.[7] Similarly, we find that the most violent acts against those who engage in same-sex behaviors occur at the same time that the same societies show their greatest intolerance for differences of religion, as well as differences in ethnicity and race. If you hate the other, you might as well hate all of the others.

DECODING OUR HISTORIES

To fully understand any written history, we have to pay close attention to the predispositions and biases of the individuals who are writing the history as well as the time in which they are writing. Certainly, as the first stories of the Iraqi war were being written, we found radically different perspectives coming from different pens within and across cultures. And it is safe to assume that as time moves on, these histories will continue to change, with most, if not all, being the truth as the writer understands it. The Arab, American, and French stories that will be spun using the same facts will be quite different. The same can be said for the stories of same-sex behaviors throughout history. We can see this when we contrast the Judeo-Christian writings that condemn homosexuality and have a virtual zero tolerance for any same-sex behavior against the perspectives offered by writers from classical Greece and the Roman Empire and throughout much of the Japanese and Chinese histories.

A telling example of how writers from different cultures use different lenses in conversing on same-sex behaviors can be found in two different bodies of literature that describe these relationships in 16th- and 17th-century Japan. Although the letters of Christian missionaries who had visited Japan were quick to denounce this part of the culture,[8] the literature written by the Japanese themselves extols the virtues of and discusses the codes that governed these relationships.[9] Not surprisingly, these literatures present clashing pictures when describing the same facts:

> In our empire of Japan **this way** [men engaged in same-gender relationships] flourished from the time of the great master Kobo. In the abbeys of Kyoto and Kamakura, and in the world of the nobles and the warriors, lovers would swear perfect and eternal love relying on no more than their mutual good will. Whether their partners were noble or common, rich or poor, was absolutely of no importance . . . In all these cases they were greatly moved by the spirit of **this way. This way** must be truly respected, and it must never be permitted to disappear, a passage taken from the 1482 work of Ijiri Chusuke, *The Essence of Jakudo.*[10] [emphasis added by Watanabe and Iwata; bracketed information added by this author]

> The abominable vice against nature [men engaged in same-gender relationships] is so popular that they [the Japanese] practice it without any feeling of shame, taken from a letter written by Saint Francis Xavier circa 1580.[11] [bracketed information added by this author]

What we learn by comparing these writings is that same-gender relationships were not unusual during this period of Japanese history, nor were they limited to particular groups within the society. We also learn that they were accepted by the Japanese themselves but, as we would expect, were viewed very differently by the Christian missionaries who came to Japan. In reading these descriptions, we also find that though Christian missionaries strongly objected to what Allessandro Valignano referred to as the "sin that will not bear mentioning,"[12] they were taken back by the overall beauty and civility of the culture. In their writings, Japan is never described as a failing or crumpling society.

In the chronicles of same-sex relationships, we find two earlier examples of possible same-sex behavior that are interesting, both of which help us to understand the importance of the filters we use in interpreting history. We draw our first example from the 1964 discovery of an Egyptian tomb constructed in the Necropolis of Saqqara circa 2400 B.C.E.[13] This particular tomb was built as the burial chamber for two Egyptians males, Niankhkhnum and Khnumhotep, both of whom served as mortuary priests and held the title of Overseer of the Manicurists in the Palace of the King, a title that typically would have been bestowed on only one individual.[14]

In uncovering the tomb, Mounir Basta, the Chief Inspector of Lower Egypt, discovered a carving of the two men embracing. Considering the rarity of any tomb built for two men, Basta, in keeping with contemporary Egypt mores, asked whether these two men were two brothers, father and son, or two officials in the king's palace, who had enjoyed a cordial friendship in life and wished to keep it after death in the nether world? The question he never asked was *whether they were lovers*—a question that would have offended his fellow Egyptians.[15]

After the initial discovery, additional sections of the tomb were uncovered and pieced together, providing even more depictions of the men in embracing positions. Upon examining these remnants in their entirety, Reeder and others noted that the multiple drawings and carvings displayed the two men in poses typically used to portray husbands and wives, hypothesizing that Niankhkhnum and Khnumhotep's relationship might be most appropriately defined as conjugal partners. In contrast, Baines, another Egyptologist, drew a different conclusion, suggesting that these men were twins and therefore buried together.[16]

In making his case for the two men being twins, even Baines uses descriptions of the multiple images of Niankhkhnum and Khnumhotep that would seem to support the argument of a same-sex relationship, including the fact that in some renderings of the two families, the men's wives were intentionally excluded: "As one moves toward the focal false doors, the owners [Niankhkhnum and Khnumhotep] cease to relate to other figures, becoming concerned with each other and the next generation, and then with each other only."[17] With the theories of same-sex relationship versus twins both contested,[18] this ongoing disagreement points to the importance of our understanding the lenses that are used by the experts who are recording and interpreting the facts for us. At one end of the spectrum, we have an expert unable or unwilling to see same-sex love portrayed in history other than in the most negative of terms. At the other extreme, we have an expert who finds ample evidence to assume same-sex attraction.

All 10 of the Chinese emperors in the Han dynasty (206 B.C.E.–1 C.E.) had male lovers, many of whom were considered men of accomplishment. In three cases the relationships between the emperor and his male partner gave rise to tales of great romantic love, the most well known being the Emperor Ai and his partner Dong Xian. Awakened from a nap, Emperor Ai was called to a meeting, but Dong Xian was still sleeping with his head on the emperor's long sleeve. Rather than disturb his partner, Ai was said to have cut off the sleeve of his robe and gone to the meeting minus the sleeve. It is reputed that to show their respect for his great affection, many of Ai's courtiers began to cut off their sleeves. The term *cut sleeve* became an appellation for male love (Crompton 2003, 214–15; Ng 1989, 77).

Our second example begins with Chinese lore. The tales of the Yellow Emperor are repeated over and over in early Chinese writings. Huang-di, the assumed first Emperor of China, ruled from 2687 to 2599 B.C.E. Throughout the stories of his life, he is credited with a host of accomplishments: the first man to study astrology as well as the inventor of the wheel and the magnet. In these stories he is also said to be the first of many Chinese emperors to include males among his sexual partners.[19]

Whether the stories in the legend of the Yellow Emperor are apocryphal or true, it comes as no surprise to scholars that he is reported to have engaged in same-sex relationships. In Chinese lore and throughout recorded Chinese history up to the early 20th century, there is a widespread acceptance of these relationships. We could therefore expect the legend of a bisexual or homosexual emperor from those who carried forward the oral tradition and the earliest written records of the Yellow Emperor. This is in keeping with their sense of nobility and accomplishment.[20] In stark contrast, we come across an almost deafening silence about the same-sex activities of our Western heroes and heroines through much of Western history, a silence that reflects a belief that any such statements might call into question the values of the time or diminish the accomplishments of these larger-than-life men and women. There are, of course, periods such as the Renaissance when the absolute silence has been broken.

Similar to the attributions credited to the Yellow Emperor, Leonardo Da Vinci is well recognized as an artist, engineer, scientist, and inventor—a man who stands as one of history's greatest minds and talents. But unlike the Yellow Emperor, Da Vinci's sexual attractions and behaviors remain an unanswered question in history (Bramly 1994; White 2000). History does tell us that there is no evidence of any romantic relationships with women and that Da Vinci surrounded himself with handsome young men, many of whom served as his models. His art and his sketches of the human anatomy also reveal his obsession with the lower physique and genitalia of the male body, an obsession that becomes even more pronounced when compared with his sparsely detailed and often incomplete drawings of women.

The only direct evidence we have of any sexual behavior on Da Vinci's part comes from an anonymous tip given to the police—a tip that accused then-17-year-old Jacopo Saltarelli of engaging in same-sex behaviors with 24-year-old Leonardo and three other codefendants. Saltarelli was rumored to be a male prostitute (Crompton 2003; Saslow 1989).

The inability to find direct and irrefutable evidence of Da Vinci's often-assumed homosexuality comes as no surprise, nor is it a particularly unique occurrence in researching the lives of famous men and women. To varying degrees, indirect evidence has been used when considering the sexual orientation of a number of his near contemporaries: Donatello, Botticelli, Michelangelo, Cellini, and Caravaggio.

THE LESSONS LEARNED

Notwithstanding the problems we face in decoding and documenting these behaviors, the available evidence provides us with a compelling, if less than complete, accounting of same-sex attraction—an accounting that offers us lessons about sexual practices and how these practices interfaced with general social interactions. Among the most significant of these are the findings that (a) same-sex behaviors have occurred throughout human history, (b) social acceptance of these behaviors is not linked to the demise or diminishment of governments or civilizations, (c) these behaviors have been expressed in a variety of ways, and (c) the expressions within a given society reflect the cultural norms of the time.

> In her 2004 biography of Florence Nightingale, Gillian Gill writes, "Let me make it clear and explicit. Florence Nightingale was not a lesbian" (p. 187). Gill makes this statement in response to suggestions that various elements in Nightingale's life and in her writings point to possible attractions to and relationships with women.
>
> In presenting the case that Nightingale was not a lesbian, Gill offers as proof of her assertion that "no one has produced any [direct] evidence that Florence Nightingale ever engaged in sexual relations with women. This I assume to be the standard working definition of lesbian" (187).
>
> The question of whether Nightingale was or was not homosexual is certainly an interesting topic for Nightingale scholars. But even more interesting are two issues that are confronted by many biographers and echoed in Gill's comments. The first of these is whether, minus unequivocal evidence, the presumption should be heterosexuality. Such sentiment often rings of an innocent-until-proven-guilty mentality, but then we must ask, guilty of what? Gill offers no evidence that Nightingale had sexual relations with a man or that she had a lifelong intimate relationship with one. Does that mean she wasn't heterosexual?
>
> The second and related issue is whether Nightingale's sexual orientation matters. The reality is that for many readers it does matter. For some the knowledge or assumption that a historic person was lesbian or gay seems to diminish or call into debate the quality of the individual's accomplishments, whereas for others it can enrich the readers' views of their own worth and potential. For which reader are we writing?

Throughout History and the Cycles of Society

Culling through the existing records, including relatively rich bodies of art and literature, over the past 35 years, scholars have been able to pen several texts describing same-sex practices throughout the development of European, Asian, and Middle Eastern cultures and in post-European-contact North and South America—chronicles that document eras marked by open acceptance and celebration as well as periods marked by scorn and punishment.[21] With considerably less documentation, anthropologists and historians have also identified direct evidence of same-sex practices among the indigenous peoples of Africa, Australia, and the inhabited islands from across the globe, as well as among Native Americans. Unfortunately, the lack of written records means that scholars have been unable to provide as much detail for these latter groups. This fact notwithstanding, it is certain that these practices predate Europeans landing on American shores, and it's often hypothesized that they extend back to the beginning of these civilizations.[22]

Within these various annals, we also find stories that predate the Babylonians and continue through to today.[23] These writings provide us with stories of great artists and philosophers as well as pictures of the Greek warriors known as the Band of Thebes, the Samurai of Japan, and Celtic warriors fighting openly with their same-sex lovers by their sides, as well as glimpses of American soldiers fighting and dying for their country while hiding their sexual identities in history's closet.

Prussian born, Baron Friedrich Wilhelm von Steuben is credited with helping George Washington organize and train the Continental army and was honored by both Washington and the U.S. Congress for his efforts. Unfortunately, what is hidden from most history books is the evidence that the Baron fled his European commission to avoid accusations about his attachment to young soldiers. When he arrived in Valley Forge, he was accompanied by his 17-year-old French interpreter. Later he adopted two handsome young American soldiers. Ironically, one month after the Baron joined Washington and his troops, another soldier, Frederick Gotthold Enslin, became the first American to be discharged from the military for same-sex behaviors (Alyson 1993).

Sergeant Leonard Matlovich received a Purple Heart and a Bronze Star for service in Vietnam. He was discharged from the Air Force when he announced publicly that he was gay. His tombstone reads, "When I was in the military, they gave me a medal for killing two men, and a discharge for loving one."

In March 2003, Eric Alva became the first American soldier to be wounded in the Iraq war, losing his leg to a land mine. Four years later, after having been praised by George Bush and Secretary Donald Rumsfeld, Eric came out as a gay American soldier and began to challenge the U.S. Defense Department's treatment of gay and lesbian members of the military.

They also offer us the personal histories of some of the most noted political leaders, economists, and scientists contrasted against the stories of unknown men and women burned at the stake during the Spanish Inquisitions and the ten thousand men who wore the pink triangle in Nazi concentration camps. Throughout the pages of history, it is made clear—same-sex practices were not limited to a few cultures or certain periods of time. Quite the contrary, these behaviors have been a universal characteristic of all societies.

The death of one man who wore the pink triangle in Hitler's concentration camps:

The loudspeakers broadcast some noisy classical music while the SS stripped him naked, shoved a tin pail over his head, and released their ferocious German Shepherds on him. The guard dogs bit into his groin and thighs; then devoured him in front of us. His shrieks of pain were distorted and amplified by the pail in which his head was trapped.

—Seel 1995, 42

Social Acceptance of Same-Sex Behavior

When we look at the total course of human history, we find that the first prohibitions against same-sex practices didn't appear until circa 630 B.C.E., when the Hebrews first posted the Holiness Codes of ritual uncleanness. (See chapter 4, "Sacred Scriptures and Homosexuality," in this text.) For most other societies, public acceptance of same-sex practices continued for centuries and, indeed, in some societies for millennia.[24] Among Native Americans and the Japanese, same-sex relationships were candidly practiced until the early and late 19th century, and among the Chinese this continued until the early 20th century, when the Communist Party placed sanctions on these practices.[25]

In commenting on the open acceptance of same-sex behaviors in past cultures, those who oppose equal rights for the LGB community frequently claim that societies that accepted homosexuality soon fell as a result of their moral decay or God's wrath. Historians on the other hand present us with quite a different chronology, one that makes clear that the acceptance

Roman laws prohibiting same-sex behaviors didn't appear until 313 C.E. under the Christian Emperor Constantine. The first Germanic prohibitions didn't occur until the 9th century C.E. And same-sex practices were common in most Native American tribes well past the first arrival of European settlers. French prohibitions of same-sex behaviors were eliminated in 1791, one year after a protest was lodged by homosexual citizens (Crompton 2003; Spencer 1995).

of same-sex behaviors has never been connected to the demise of a culture or nation state. This is well illustrated by the fact that the Roman Empire did not fall during the notorious rein of the pagan emperors Caligula or Nero, but only after 150 years of rule by the Christian emperors. Likewise, although same-sex behaviors were accepted for more than a millennium throughout early and classic Greece, when the Greeks were finally conquered, they were defeated by the Macedonians, who were also engaged in same-sex practices. And as noted previously, the first 10 emperors of the Han dynasty, who led China through one of its most productive epochs, were among the numerous Chinese emperors to have male partners.[26]

Richard Nixon provided a classic, albeit somewhat inebriated, example of this distorted historic narrative:

Do you know what happened to the Romans? The last six Roman emperors were fags: the last six. Nero had a public wedding to a boy. [unintelligible] You know that. You know what happened to the Popes? It's all right that, po-po-Popes were laying the nuns, that's been going on for years, centuries, but, when the popes, when the Catholic Church went to hell, in, I don't know, three or four centuries ago, it was homosexual. And finally it had to be cleaned out.

Now, that's what's happened to Britain, it happened earlier to France. And let's look at the strong societies. The Russians—God damn it, they root them out; they don't let them around at all. You know what I mean?

I don't know what they do with them. . . . You see homosexuality, dope, immorality in general: These are the enemies of strong societies.

—As taken from audiotapes in the Oval Office, quoted in Gardner 2006

Of course, Nixon's history was completely wrong. Most of the emperors from Constantine forward were Christians and, as best we know, heterosexuals.

In stark contrast to the spurious link between the decline of civilization and the acceptance of same-sex behaviors, we find that the greatest persecutions of homosexuals and bisexuals occurred during periods considered among the worst examples of human oppression and intolerance, including the Valencian Inquisition, Hitler's Germany, Stalin's rein in the Soviet Union, and the Islamic fundamentalist states of today. During these eras, individuals who engaged in same-sex relationships were subjected to being burned at the stake in the name of God, being treated as the most despised of the prisoners in the concentration camps, and being jailed as enemies of the state in Soviet gulags. We also encounter similar, albeit less onerous, patterns of persecution during some of the darker periods in societies such as ours. A notable example of this occurred during the U.S. Senate hearings in the 1950s when Senator McCarthy, Roy Cohen (McCarthy's assistant, who was regarded as a closeted gay man), and FBI Director J. Edgar Hoover (who is also thought to have been a closeted gay man) leveled charges of sexual deviance against numbers of individuals.[27] Although it would be an error for us to conclude that the acceptance of same-sex behaviors always heralded the best of human civilizations, it is by no means an overstatement when we assert that the persecution of same-sex behaviors is strongly linked to societal oppression and intolerance.

Some gay men and lesbians have sought liberation in what turned out to be the most oppressive of governments. Henry Hay and Michel Foucault, icons in the gay and queer rights movements, believed that communism was a path to liberation, and Gertrude Stein supported Hitler and fascism during the beginning of Hitler's reign.

> Obviously, being extremely bright and homosexual doesn't inoculate you against poor political judgments, just as being bright and heterosexual doesn't prevent poor judgment.

Different Expressions of Same-Sex Attraction

Throughout human civilization we find a range of same-sex practices, both homosexual and bisexual. At times these expressions of same-sex attraction seem familiar to those we find in today's society, and at other times, we are apt to be taken back and may feel uncomfortable with particular behaviors. When looking at these differences, it's important that we understand them in their cultural context, the same as we do when we look at historic heterosexual practices such as polygamy and incest.

> History provides too few recorded examples of homosexuality and bisexuality among females—that is, until women began to exert their rights. As this happened, more and more stories of lesbian and bisexual relationships among female thought leaders emerged. During the late 19th century and early 20th century, women such as Jane Addams, one of the first women to win the Noble Peace Prize; Virginia Wolf, author; Isadora Duncan, famed dancer; and Gertrude Stein, author, were playing an increasingly important role in American and European culture. And with this came greater attention to their personal lives (Benstock 1989; Newton 1989).

The stories of the past provide a picture of adults focused exclusively on the same-gender partners (homosexual) as well as adults who engaged in same-gender relationships and opposite-gender marriages, simultaneously or at differing times in their lives (bisexual). In most historic records we come across more illustrations of same-gender relationships among men than among women. We can't be certain to what degree this was a result of actual greater prevalence of these practices among men, as current statistics would support, or an artifact of a history that too often ignores women and their roles in society.

In examining these patterns closely, we realize that the differing expressions of and attitudes about same-sex behavior reflected other social constructs of the time. In societies where women were treated as property, adult males who assumed the receptive or passive role in same-sex relationships tended to be ridiculed, whereas the active or assertive partner escaped such censure. In cultures that accepted males and females when they adopted different gender identities, men who assumed the receptive or passive role in a same-gender relationship were respected and at times honored as being two-spirited.

In a number of Native American tribes, young boys who showed no inclination to engage in male-centered activities were encouraged to join in with the women, adopting a new gender identity that was accepted by the tribe. As they grew older, many of these men would enter into marriages with other males who were inclined to same-gender attraction but who practiced the more traditional tribal roles. In several of these tribes, two-spirited men were also seen as shamans or holy men, engaging in ritualistic ceremonies. This practice of allowing young boys to choose a different gender identity was also an accepted practice among numerous island cultures, including the Tanala of Madagascar.

Among the Arandas of Australia, it was common for young adult males to take younger male partners as their "wives," living together until the older of the two came of age to marry a woman. Similar practices have also been recorded among the Keraki of New Guinea and native Haitians. Although there are fewer such examples, same-sex relationships among women have been noted is several of these cultures as well, including among the Arandas of Australia and some Native American tribes in which women might pursue the life of a warrior.

Sexual and romantic relationships between older males were ridiculed at various times in Greek and Roman history, as in the case of Julius Caesar's affair with King Nicomedes of Bithynia. The negative feelings toward such relationships arose from a belief that an adult male who assumed a passive role in sex was likely to do the same in his political life. This certainly was not true in Julius Caesar's case (Williams 1999).

Many of our contemporary discussions on the history of same-sex behaviors have focused on early and classic Greece as well as on the Roman

Republic and Empire, but there are compelling works of art and rich bodies of literature demonstrating that same-sex relationships were openly accepted and even honored through two thousand years of Chinese and Japanese history, up until the late 19th and early 20th centuries. In each of these societies, we have records that provide us with different voices from within the culture, voices that offer multiple perspectives on same-sex behaviors. And in each instance we can also track changes in the behaviors and attitudes across time, suggesting that it would be naïve to assume that any single snapshot can be used to characterize the total history of same-sex behavior within these civilizations. Nonetheless, we see patterns that help us understand how same-sex practices reflect the customs of the time.

Some of the more notable examples of same-sex attractions among women come from the poetry and songs of Sappho, a 7th-century B.C.E. citizen of the Isle of Lesbos:

> He seems as fortunate as the gods to me, the man who sits opposite you and listens nearby to your sweet voice and lovely laughter. Truly that sets my heart trembling in my breast. For when I look at you for a moment, then it is no longer possible for me to speak; my tongue has snapped, at once a subtle fire has stolen beneath my flesh, I see nothing with my eyes, my ears hum, sweat pours from me, a trembling seizes me all over, I am greener than grass, and it seems to me that I am little short of dying.

> —Sappho, as quoted in Crompton 2003, 17

At one point exiled in Sicily for her political activism, Sappho eventually returned to her native Isle of Lesbos to become a doyen for a band of younger women who shared her views and tastes. The honors shown to Sappho through memorialization in statutes and paintings and the fact that her writings have survived suggest that at least some Greeks were sympathetic to her work and her views.

The patriarchy found throughout much of the history of these four societies is made apparent in the availability of information on the practice of same-sex behaviors. Although male and female same-sex practices are recorded in all four, the disparity in the attention paid and the honor given to male behaviors in contrast to the relative absence of mention of female behaviors mirrors the male dominance in these cultures. The attention to male sexuality in general and male same-sex behaviors in particular, though certainly not unique to these civilizations, becomes most obvious when we compare it to the attention given to female sexuality in some early matriarchal cultures.[28] However, as humans moved from matriarchies to male-dominated societies, women's sexuality became less of a focus and was often ignored or denied or, at times, strictly limited and controlled.

Evidence documents that same-sex behaviors have taken various forms resonating with other cultural norms. The age differences in the commonly accepted adult male and adolescent boy pairings in classic Greek culture were not that dissimilar from the accepted age difference between husbands and wives.[29] And on many occasions these age differences were less than those found among married couples, where husbands in their thirties would marry girls in their mid-teens.

Similarly, strong biases opposing same-sex interactions among women but allowing them among men are most frequently traced to periods of greater cultural misogyny. And instances of hidden expressions of same-gender affection can be linked to periods of the most stringent political or religious sanctions.

20TH- AND 21ST-CENTURY HISTORIES

When many of us think of the history of homosexuality and same-sex behavior, we tend to focus on ancient cultures, forgetting 20th-century history. We have heard the stories of Rome and Greece in public folklore, but our understanding of today's issues is too often limited to the headlines on same-sex marriage. Most of us have no idea of how we got to where we are on this topic. Nor do we know how gay men, lesbians, and bisexuals have influenced other key stories in our contemporary history. The material is not covered in our texts, our teachers don't know this part of our cultural history, our K–12 schools think of these stories as too controversial, and our colleges don't see it as central to their mission. But these reactions don't come from any lack of a history to be told.

We open our textbooks and read about the race riots of the 1960s and 1970s, but with few exceptions,[30] we don't read anything about Stonewall, the 1969 riot that is credited as the beginning of what has become the gay and lesbian rights movement. Nor do we learn about the gay rights movement in San Francisco. Why would we think it important to educate ourselves about the origins of the issues that dominate so many of today's elections?

When we study black history, we learn about the Harlem Renaissance, a period of incredible artistic accomplishment among blacks in New York. We also study the many accomplishments of Martin Luther King Jr. These and related events are important to giving voice to the African Americans who helped shape today's culture and society and to providing the faces we can identify with if we ourselves are African American. But we don't learn that Langston Hughes, Zora Neale Hurston, Ethel Waters, and James Weldon Johnson were homosexual or bisexual. Nor do we learn or teach that Bayard Rustin—the man who introduced and tutored Martin Luther King on Gandhi, helped King found the Southern Christian Leadership Conference, and served as the main architect for the 1963 March on Washington—was gay and was asked to step down from his leadership position when Senator Strom Thurman and J. Edgar Hoover threatened to denounce King for his involvement with a known homosexual. Why would we want LGB African American students to know about the proud heritage from which they came?

We read about the Holocaust because it's important for us to learn about the horrendous atrocities one group can inflict on another. And it's important that those of us who are Jewish understand an incredibly painful part of our history. But it doesn't seem important that those of us who are gay understand the thriving gay culture that existed in Berlin prior to Hitler's rise to power, as well as the fact that many young gay men joined the Jews in the gas chambers?

Our headlines focus on the environmental movement, and many of us know the historic importance of Rachel Carson's 1962 book *Silent Spring* in getting this movement started, but do we know that she was a lesbian? And does she provide a role model for the young girl in Topeka who is just discovering her own sexual orientation?

The women's movement has reshaped our culture, opening up doors for women in the board room, the science laboratory, the church pulpit, and the halls of government. But do our daughters know that the campaign that gave them the right to vote was first spearheaded by a woman who was most likely a lesbian, Susan B. Anthony? And that many of the women who followed Anthony's footsteps in seeking women's rights were homosexual and bisexual? Or do we hide these facts in the deep recesses of history, allowing heterosexual women to feel comfortable distancing themselves from their lesbian sisters?

There are so many rich and profound historic stories of homosexuals and bisexuals within our own contemporary cultures. But these stories are usually confined to single-topic textbooks—*Hidden from History: Reclaiming the Gay and Lesbian Past;*[31] *A History of Homosexuality*[32]—and rarely if ever included in the general histories of North and South America, Europe, Asia, Africa, and Australia. The fact that these stories aren't in these books isn't because they aren't important or because no one knows about them. It is essentially censorship—it is *too controversial* to tell the true story, so let's leave it on the cutting room floor.

It will be interesting to watch how the histories of the early 21st century are written. With the focus placed on gay and lesbian rights and other issues related to homosexuality, it seems improbable that our general textbooks can maintain their embargo on discussing this topic. But will the voices heard in the textbooks extend back in time, and will the faces seen within these pages document the incredible and typically untold accomplishments of homosexuals and bisexuals throughout history?

STRAIGHT TALK

With the prehistoric and historic evidence we have, it's safe to assume that same-sex behaviors have been an integral part of human culture since homo sapiens first walked this planet. Whether it is named or not, the same is likely to be true for homosexuality (i.e., the exclusive attraction to people of the same sex). The men who have practiced these behaviors have thrived in some societies and have been scorned and tortured in others. Too often the women who have engaged in these behaviors have been completely hidden from history.

Although there is no doubt that these behaviors have occurred during some of the most licentious of times, the fact is that so has heterosexuality. Heterosexual and homosexual behaviors occur during times of war and in times of peace, when we have abundance and when we have famine, when our governments are open and when they are repressive—one thing you can pretty well count on is that humans engage in sex, be they heterosexual, homosexual, or bisexual. That being said, it is also true that the way we express our sexuality is influenced by the societies in which we live. Do we tend to have one partner or multiple partners; are we open about our sexuality, or do we hide in a closet; do we commit to lifelong relationships at 15 or at 25; do we couple with partners of the same age, or do we take on partners younger or older than ourselves? All of these are influenced by the cultural mores of the time.

Another fact of history is that those societies that have been the most repressive are the same societies that have been the most hostile to homosexuality. And those societies that have been most remarkable have been to greater or lesser degree the most accepting of same-sex attraction. The thought that governments have failed because they began accepting homosexuality is based on terribly flawed reasoning and very bad historical analyses. Ironically, Rome didn't fall when it embraced homosexuality; it fell after it passed laws condemning same-sex behaviors. Rome accepted same-sex behaviors at its zenith, as did Greece, Japan, China, and Native American cultures. The most shameful periods of Christianity are the same periods when homosexuals were burned at the stake.

Homosexuals and bisexuals have made and continue to make significant contributions to world history. Those cultures that have been the most accepting of same-sex behaviors and that have the best written records provide us with a rich and open understanding of the numerous accomplishments of the elite males of the era who engaged in same-sex practices. When we search the records of repressive cultures, we are forced to discover homosexuality through innuendo and circumstantial evidence. But the evidence is there if we are willing to piece it together. As we have discovered throughout this text, until recently, the lives of women who engaged in same-sex practices have been too often hidden in history, less because of homophobia and more so because of misogynic attitudes in societies.

In speaking to different well-educated groups of heterosexuals, bisexuals, and homosexuals, one other fact becomes painfully apparent. Most of the men and women I speak to know a lot about the current debates on sexual orientation, but very few know anything about the history of same-sex behaviors, and some who claim they do have quite distorted pictures of this history. The old Soviet Union could not have done a better job of censoring their textbooks than the West has done when it comes to this part of our history.

NOTES

1. TFP Committee on American Issues 2004.
2. Ehrlich 2002; Ford and Beach 1951; Crompton 2003; Schalow 1989.
3. Vasey 1995.
4. Greenberg 1988.
5. Ehrlich 2002; Ford and Beach 1951; Katz 1976; Muscarella 2002.
6. Boswell 1980; Crompton 2003; Ng 1989.
7. Hubbard 2003 Massey 1988.
8. Crompton 2003.

9. Schalow 1989.

10. As quoted in Watanabe and Iwata 1989, 19.

11. As quoted in Watanabe and Iwata 1989, 20.

12. Crompton 2003, 412.

13. Reeder 2000.

14. Baines 1985.

15. As cited in Reeder 2000 193.

16. Baines 1985.

17. Baines 1985, 466.

18. Wilford 2005.

19. Crompton 2003.

20. Crompton 2003; Ng 1989.

21. Boswell 1990; Crompton 2003; Duberman, Vicinus, and Chauncey 1989; Hinsch 1990; Hubbard 2002; Panate 2006; Spencer 1999.

22. Aldrich 2006; Ford and Beach 1951; Katz 1976; Spencer 1995; Wallace 2006.

23. Boswell 1990; Crompton 2003; Duberman, Vicinus, and Chauncey 1989; Hinsch 1990; Hubbard 2002; Panate 2006; Spencer 1995

24. Boswell 1980; Crompton 2003; Spencer 1995.

25. Crompton 2003; Hinsch 1990; Ng 1989; Schalow 1989; Spencer 1995; Watanabe and Iwata 1989.

26. Crompton 2003; Hinsch 1990; Ng 1989; Schalow 1989; Spencer 1995.

27. Katz 1976; Spencer 1995.

28. Spencer 1995.

29. Hubbard 2002; Massey 1988.

30. Boyer, Clark, Hawley, Kett, Salisbury, Sitkoff, and Woloch 2004, 913.

31. Dode 2004.

32. Duberman, Vicinus, and Chauncey 1989.

7

Pardon Me, But Do You Have Size 13 Toe Shoes in Stock?

I can't remember how I ended up home alone that spring evening, but I do remember the fear that raced through my 15-year-old body when I answered the doorbell to find Tim, a 17-year-old who sat behind me in history, and two of his friends at the front door. What in the world would have made Tim believe it was okay for him to bring these two 18- or 19-year-olds with makeup on their faces to my parents' house? My god, what would have happened if either of my parents or one of my siblings had answered the door? What would the neighbors say if they saw these two patently obvious gay males standing on our porch talking to me? Having been born well before every other television show and movie had a sympathetic gay or lesbian included in the cast, I wondered about my own future—were these examples of the man I was destined to become? All of these thoughts were racing through my adolescent brain as these three stood in front of me—my first face-to-face confrontation with the hyper-effeminate stereotype of the homosexual male. Although I was beginning to understand that I was gay, I wasn't ready to face this. No, I didn't want to go for a ride with them; what I wanted to do was find a place to hide from them, from my family, and probably from myself. I was petrified and horrified.

Over the course of the next several years, I was to meet an ever-increasing number of gay and lesbian stereotypes—the unmarried male school teacher who dressed impeccably well, always had a smile and kind word, and while maintaining all of the appropriate boundaries, honestly listened to my coming-out traumas; the working-class lesbian couple who took me to the firing range for rifle practice, something I wasn't particularly good at; the married mainline Protestant minister who made me uncomfortable; the science teacher who lived with her partner, a principle in the school district next to ours; and so on and so on. My catalog of homosexual stereotypes was ever-expanding, growing at the same rate and with the same complexities and contradictions as my catalog of heterosexual stereotypes—for example, the straight woman who worked hard at being a great mother versus the straight woman who slapped and screamed at her children in the grocery store.

In building my schema for organizing these various groups, I was more than happy to incorporate the many positive stereotypes of the gay male—well dressed, talented, and well educated. But I remained very uncomfortable with the stereotypes of the screaming gay man who used female pronouns when he referred to other men—"Isn't she something?"—or the lonely and mentally unstable gay man. These were the ones most denigrated by society and therefore the men I desperately didn't want to become. Of course, I had no problem with creating compartments for the intolerant and illiterate heterosexual. In some ways those stereotypes gave me some comfort and a false sense of superiority—"You may think I am strange, but at least I dress well, and I am not a bigot," which of course I was, as proven by that very thought.

As I was honing my gaydar (i.e., the skill of identifying individuals as gay or lesbian), I ran across a number of cases that would punch holes in one or another of the sieves I was using to sort people—the two gay hog farmers, the lesbian runway model, the effeminate yet aggressively heterosexual music professor. At times, it seemed I was finding almost as many exceptions as I was people who fit my various rules. There was an ample number of lesbians who were great athletes, but there were also female athletes who weren't lesbians, and God bless my friend Georgia—she couldn't hit a tennis ball, golf ball, or softball to save her soul. Of course, I couldn't either, but that didn't run counter to the stereotype. I met plenty of artistic gay men, but I met even more gay guys who had no talent whatsoever, and their sense of home décor and the clothes they wore showed it.

Despite all of the exceptions, I didn't spend a lot of time thinking about the accuracy of the traits I was using to sort straight from gay or about the origins of these traits. Were these characteristics innately tied to the person's sexual orientation, were they behaviors fostered by societal expectations or pressures, or were they mechanisms the individuals chose or cultivated as a way of fitting into one group or opting out of another?

Although I was oblivious to these questions, I couldn't ignore the differences between my list and the lists being used by individuals who thought the world might be better off without me and my tribe. My list placed a lot more emphasis on the positive traits than some of the lists of family and neighbors. I saw the world as more beautiful and creative and as more open and accepting thanks to my gay brothers and lesbian sisters. Others saw my friends and me as troubled individuals, people who would be lonely and hidden in the corners of society. And still others saw the world as in danger of moral decay or total collapse because of us. So whose accounting was right—which if any characteristics distinguished the homosexual from the heterosexual? And would society be better or worse off if my friends and I disappeared? Or maybe there were no real differences or at least none of cosmic consequence.

As I considered the different lists we were all using, it became apparent that even when the attributes on our various lists were the same, our attitudes about these characteristics could be quite different—"he dances so well" might become "he's so gay" or "he's such a faggot." "She can play ball" can easily morph into "she's such a lesbo" or into "what a bull dyke." In other instances we associated very different qualities with being gay or lesbian. In my various images of the gay male, I would see my friend Ron, an incredibly talented kindergarten teacher, inspiring his students to explore their ever-expanding world; others might see the priest who abused young altar boys, taking their innocence from them. How did we come to construct these different homosexualities?

WHY OUR DIFFERENT PICTURES OF HOMOSEXUALITY

Although queer theorists might be missing a major part of the answer as to why some of us are homosexual and others of us are not—or for that matter they may not even understand what the question means—they do offer us a lot to think about when we consider how we as humans express and construct our images of homosexuality in our individual lives and throughout our many cultures. When our culture sees homosexuality as a threat to social order, it almost always associates same-sex love with other culturally threatening behaviors; when civilization accepts same-sex love, the men and women who engage in these relationships will often be celebrated. We know that today many fundamentalist Muslims see homosexuality as one more manifestation of the evil influence of the Western infidel, yet in the eighth century, St. Boniface was more than ready to believe that the successful Muslim invasion of the Iberian Peninsula was, at least in part, due to Christians succumbing to the evils of same-sex love practiced by Arabs of the time.[1] Standing in stark contrast to linking homosexuality to the per-ceived evils of the day, among Native American tribes across both conti-nents, two-spirit people (homosexuals) were often elevated to the position of healers and prophets.[2] For some of us, homosexuals were the voice and hands of God, whereas for others, gays and lesbians have been the instru-ments of the devil. For Nazis, homosexuality was a sign of societal and mil-itary weakness, whereas in Ancient Greece, there were those who felt that an army or a government of same-sex lovers could bring upon a utopia of sorts. Depending on where and when you were born, you would be offered very different perspectives on homosexuality. (See chapter 6, "The Down-fall of Society," and its discussion of the Sacred Band of Thebes.)

Following are two very different views on how homosexuality affects the strength of a nation:

Those who are considering love between men or between women are our enemies. Anything that emasculates our people and makes us fair game for our enemies we reject. . . . History teaches us a different les-son: Might makes right. And the stronger will always prevail against the weaker. Today we are the weaker. Let us make sure that we will become the stronger again! This we can do only if we exercise moral restraint. Therefore, we reject all immorality, especially love between men.

—Quoted in a 1937 statement from Hitler's National
Socialist Party, as cited in Haeberle 1981, 282

And if there were only some way of contriving that a state or an army should be made up of lovers and their loves, they would be the very best governors of their own city, abstaining from all dishonor, and emu-lating one another in honor; and when fighting at each other's side, although a mere handful, they would overcome the world. For what lover would not choose rather to be seen by all mankind than by his beloved, either abandoning his post or throwing away his arms? He would rather die a thousand deaths rather than endure this. Or who would desert his beloved or fail him in the hour of danger?

—Phaedrus speech in Plato's Symposium,
found in Crompton 2003, 3

But when we look at a particular culture, we need to be careful to not assume that the prevailing view is singular and absolute; if we dig deeper we are likely to find divergent and dissenting voices. In the Boor's Tale, a Japanese manuscript written in the 1600s, which was a period of relative openness, two young men spend the night comparing the virtues of the Way of Youth (same-sex love) to the Way of Women (heterosexual love). In their dialogue each extols the virtues of his own sexual preference and attacks the virtues of the other: "The youth's elegant form . . . is like the willow tree bending in the wind" versus "My image of a boy fanatic . . . He doesn't cut his nails and his hair is as reddish and wild as that of an orangutan."[3] In *An Underground Life: Memoirs of a Gay Jew in Nazi Berlin,* Gad Beck allows us to peer into the souls of those men who were somewhat open in expressing their homosexuality even while ten thousand men wearing pink triangles were joining the millions of Jews being sent to Hitler's extermination camps: "Manfred and I were a couple; all our friends knew. I made sure Mamsi met him too. . . . The fact that she liked him immediately made me feel all the more in love and helped me forget all the many problems."[4] In any given culture, you will find individuals carrying diverging images of homosexuality, at times holding on to the past and at other times foreshadowing the future.

In examining how and why we hold so many diverging views on homosexuality, it's important that we're careful not to assume that relationship means cause and effect—a tendency we have had to fight against in interpreting much of the research we have been examining throughout this book. Does John hold conservative views on homosexuality because the church he goes to teaches these, or does he go to this particular church because he holds conservative views? Or maybe, he holds conservative views about homosexuality and goes to a conservative church because that's what his parents taught him, and that's where they took him every Sunday? Which is the cause and which is the effect?

Throughout many parts of Europe and the Western hemisphere attitudes about homosexuality have been shifting over the past several decades. In 1978, 53 percent of Americans believed that homosexuals should have equal employment rights contrasted against 33 percent who felt they shouldn't. By 2008 these numbers had changed dramatically—89 percent of Americans felt that gay men and lesbians should hold equal employment rights, with only 9 percent opposing these rights—a very vocal 9 percent. Possibly even more telling is the fact that in 1978, 14 percent of respondents declared themselves as undecided, but in 2008 the number of undecided respondents had dropped to 2 percent of the total.[5] We find similar attitudinal changes on questions about legality versus illegality of same-sex behavior between consenting adults and recognition of homosexual relationships, although the shifts on these latter topics are not as dramatic as on employment discrimination. As time moves on, fewer of us are sitting on the fence, and we are becoming more open to lesbians and gay men in our society. But we are far from being a totally accepting society. When it comes to support for marriage, in 2008, 56 percent of Americans still opposed legalizing marriage, and we were at a 48–48 percent tie on whether homosexuality was morally right.

But the degree of change in attitudes has not been the same across all borders, with the United States moving more slowly than our neighbors to the north and most of them to the south.[6] In the spring of 2007, the Pew Research Group conducted a survey of 47 nations from around the world, finding that 49 percent of U.S. citizens said that homosexuality is a way of life that should be accepted by society, compared to 41 percent who felt that it shouldn't. In Canada these numbers were 70 to 21 percent; in Argentina the numbers were 72 to 21 percent; and in Chile they were 64 to 31 percent. Only two of the Western hemisphere countries out of the eight surveyed fell below U.S. acceptance levels. These were Venezuela (47% acceptable within society to 50% unacceptable) and Bolivia (44% acceptable within society to 49% unacceptable).[7]

Examining the results of the Pew survey from across the Atlantic, we can see that Europe has continued to have a lavender curtain that very closely follows the same geographic borders of the old iron curtain. In 2007, rates of accepting homosexuality tracked at 86, 83, 82, 81, 71, and 65 percent for Sweden, France, Germany, England, and Italy, respectively. In contrast, the rates of acceptance in the Ukraine, Russia, and Poland tracked at 19, 20, and 45 percent, respectively. In the Czech Republic and Slovakia, acceptance rates were 83 and 66 percent. Having a Slovak and Polish heritage, I have mixed feelings about my cousins across the sea.

Using results from the same survey, we find the greatest opposition to homosexuality occurs in Africa and the Middle East, with Egypt and Mali holding the dubious distinction of only 1 percent of their respective populations believing that homosexuality should be accepted within society. Ethiopia and Nigeria come in second from the bottom with 2 percent acceptance rates. Iran was not included among the Middle Eastern countries surveyed.

So what do we know about current worldviews on homosexuality? We know that societal acceptance of homosexuality runs the full gamut. In some European countries, 80 percent or more of the population find it to be a perfectly acceptable lifestyle. On the complete other end of the spectrum, 85 percent or more of the populations in Africa and the Middle East see homosexuality as an unacceptable way of life, with the exception of South Africa and Lebanon. With 49 percent of its population declaring homosexuality as an acceptable lifestyle, in 2007 the United States had the lowest acceptance level of any Western industrialized nation.

Employing the Pew Research Center's data for its 2007 survey, I was able to run a set of correlations to see what if any significant relationships existed between national response rates on the question of acceptance of homosexuality and attitudes about (a) the role of men and women in political life, (b) how belief in God affects morality, and (c) the quality of life within the country. When looking at opinions on men and women's ability to serve as political leaders, survey results indicate that the more likely a nation was to rate homosexuality as an acceptable way of life, the more likely it was to see men and women as equally qualified to hold political office ($r = .77$, $df = 46$, $p < .0001$). Populations that felt that homosexuality was less acceptable as a way of life were overwhelmingly more likely to see men as better political leaders ($r = .71$, $df = 46$, $p < .0001$). In countries where people told the Pew researchers it was necessary to believe in God to lead a moral life, they also told the researchers that homosexuality was an unacceptable way of life ($r = .77$, $df = 46$, $p < .0001$). And those populations that felt a person could be moral and have good values even if she or he didn't believe in God were more likely to accept homosexuality ($r = .78$, $df = 46$, $p < .0001$). When religious freedom registered as the most important concern in an individual's life, these individuals were significantly less likely to see homosexuality as an acceptable way of life ($r = -70$, $d = 46$, $p < .0001$). Finally, people who saw their lives as the best possible lives they could have were more likely to believe homosexuality was an acceptable way of life ($r = .76$, $df = 46$, $p < .0001$), whereas populations that saw their lives as being less than they should be were more likely to see homosexuality as unacceptable ($r = .49$, $df = 46$, $p < .0001$).

When we look at countries from across the globe, we also find that the people who are most concerned about their right to practice their religion are the same people who see homosexuality as an unacceptable way of life. The same populations were also less likely to believe that women could govern as well as men, and they were less satisfied with the quality of their lives.

In looking at differences within European countries, Stulhofer and Rimac found that homonegativity was also related to gross domestic product (GDP) and the urbanization of the country. The greater the economic development and urbanization in a given country, the less likely you would find homonegativity among the population.[8]

Individual Views

If GDP, urbanization, religious beliefs, political systems, and general satisfaction with life are predictors of how a nation rejects or accepts homosexuality, what variables do we use to predict the individual citizen's view? Not surprisingly, the variables are similar to the predictors of societal attitudes. But before we look at the particular characteristics that are related to individual perceptions of homosexuality, we should note that individual perceptions don't fall into simple dichotomous categories of accept versus reject but are much more multifaceted. We might even think of our attitudes about homosexuality as a game of Twister, where one of our legs could be on one point on the floor mat (homosexuals should not be discriminated against in employment) while our other foot (homosexuals should not be able to serve openly in the military) and our two arms (gay men are too promiscuous; lesbians are remarkable athletes) could be on completely different markers. Our appendages might be squarely lined up on the mat, or they might have us slightly off-balance.

Andrew Sullivan, a politically conservative gay writer, suggests that different elements of our individual beliefs about homosexuality might be located at different points along a continuum that extends from prohibitionist on one end to liberationist on the other, with conservative and liberal beliefs falling in between.[9] For the prohibitionists, homosexuality is a moral transgression too heinous to be tolerated within the society. The conservative accepts that homosexuals exist but feels this is a matter of private conduct and doesn't need to be dealt with in public forums or through laws. The liberal, on the other hand, assumes that homosexuals should have all of the legal rights of the heterosexual and expects the homosexual to assume the same moral postures expected of heterosexuals. And finally, the liberationist (queer theorist) asserts that our social rules need to be changed and prohibitions lifted for all humans: people who choose to be intimate with members of the same sex have no need or reason to explain these behaviors or to fit them into some constructed social norms (e.g., monogamous or "age-appropriate" relationships).

N.E. Walls provides us with an alternative way of understanding our perspectives on homosexuality—degrees of bias expressed through differing stereotypes.[10] In developing his Multidimensional Heterosexism Inventory, Walls identified four different categories of prejudice about homosexuality: positive stereotypic heterosexism, paternalistic heterosexism, amnestic heterosexism, and aversive heterosexism. We can probably assume a fifth category—that of the individual who sees no differences among heterosexuals and homosexuals. Those of us who hold a positive bias see lesbians and gay men as having some preferred attributes—for example, lesbian are better at camping and fishing when compared to heterosexual women. The picture may be positive, but we still differentiate homosexuals from heterosexuals. If we are paternalistic in our views, we would not want our children to be homosexual, ostensibly to protect them from the intolerance they could face in society. Those of us who are amnestic deny the prejudices that continue to confront homosexuals, claiming that gays and lesbians can be full participating members in today's society and have all the protections and rights they need. And if we hold aversive views, we feel that lesbians and gay men have become too radical in their demands.

The models by Walls and Sullivan provide two frameworks for conceptualizing the variations in our attitudes about homosexuals and homosexuality. Their works also suggest that people can and do shift positions over time. But their models are not confined to straight men and women's views about same-sex relationships. Gay men, lesbians, and bisexuals can exhibit traits associated with any one of these categories, moving over time from one to another or in some cases becoming locked into a set of beliefs. We certainly know from the research on ex-gay ministries that some gay men, lesbians, and bisexuals see their own homosexuality through the lenses of a prohibitionist or aversive heterosexist, causing them great conflict in their sense of self-worth. My own experience suggests to me that it's likely that more gay men and women fall under Sullivan's liberal category, but there are certainly a noticeable number of homosexuals and bisexuals who live their lives closeted, echoing the sentiments found in Sullivan's conservative category, with the smallest but very vocal contingency identifying themselves as liberationists. However, there is no solid research to support that my personal experience provides a particularly accurate depiction.

Now, back to the question we started with—what variables are good indicators of our personal attitudes about homosexuality? The research strongly suggests that if we are heterosexual, we are more likely to be accepting of bisexuals and homosexuals when we have close friends or family members who are themselves gay, lesbian, or bisexual. Women are also more likely to be accepting than are men, and when females hold stereotypes about gay men or lesbians, the stereotypes tend to be more positive in nature. And finally, women are more likely to have close relationships with gay men or lesbians.[11] After all, it's fun to go shopping with gay men. But lest we forget, correlation doesn't necessarily mean cause.

· So does a close relationship cause greater acceptance, or does greater acceptance allow you to develop close relationships? Or is this a synergistic connection—acceptance breeds friendship, which breeds greater acceptance? Or it could be friendship breeds acceptance, which opens you up to even more friendships. Or maybe being a woman means you are more nurturing and thus more accepting and willing to build friendships. Was it the chicken, the egg, or the genetic code found in the rooster that started it all?

Age is also a predictor of acceptance levels, with the older among us being the least accepting. Of course, this doesn't mean that all older people have problems with accepting homosexuality, as clearly demonstrated by some of the sweetest members of my family—my now-sainted aunts. Nor does this correlation between age and attitudes about homosexuality mean that cultural changes occur only among the younger members of our society. In a study comparing Canadian and U.S. acceptance levels, Andersen and Fetner[12] examined and reported on acceptance levels in the two countries from 1981 to 2000. As part of their analyses, these researchers looked at how different birth cohorts viewed homosexuality over the two decades. On a 1 to 10 scale, with 10 being completely accepting and 1 expressing low tolerance, U.S. citizens born before 1920 ranked their tolerance level at 1.82 in 1981. They were 60 years or older at the time. In 2000, U.S. citizens from this same birth cohort, who were now 80 years or older, ranked their tolerance level at 2.41. Canadian citizens in the same birth cohort began with an acceptance ranking at 1.81 in 1981; by 2000 these citizens, at 80+ years old, rated their tolerance levels at 3.74. U.S. citizens who were 18–20 years old reported acceptance levels at 2.72 in 1981. In 2000, when they were 37 to 39 years old, their average tolerance level had climbed to 4.96, almost halfway to total acceptance. Canadian citizens who were in the same birth cohort reported an average tolerance level of 3.54 in 1981; this had changed to 5.98 by 2000. Age and the passage of time both make a difference in our views about homosexuality. Over time both older and younger people are changing their minds, but younger members of society are starting out as more accepting.

Exposure to media may be one variable that accounts for changes in attitudes. In one study, Levina, Waldo, and Fitzgerald (2000) documented that two weeks after seeing either a negative media presentation on homosexuality or a positive and sympathetic depiction, the people who watched the negative film and those that watched the positive film had significantly different responses when asked questions about homosexuality that were hidden in a seemingly unrelated survey.

Religious beliefs and practices are other strong predictors of our views on homosexuality, with those of us from conservative faiths and those of us who attend church/synagogue/mosque expressing more negative opinions on homosexuality. The same is true about our political affiliations; the more conservative we are politically, the greater the probability that we will show bias against homosexuals and bisexuals.[13] In this case, cause-and-effect hypotheses can be somewhat tricky. Does my church dictate my beliefs, or do my beliefs determine the church to which I go or don't go? Or do the two feed off of each other? The correlation among these variables also raises an interesting question of how I handle conflict between church or political doctrine and personal codes of morality—do I leave the church or my political party, change my belief system, or sit by quietly, ignoring the conflict, like so many Catholics who have had the vasectomy or are taking the pill and so many Log Cabin Republicans do when their candidates votes on gay rights issues? I have friends who use each of these techniques to handle discord between personal beliefs and religious or political views. In some cases I have seen this discord cause terrible psychic trauma that is replayed over and over in their lives.

We also find studies that show a correlation between race and bias against homosexuals, with African Americans reporting higher levels of negative views.[14] Once again, there is a significant difference between male and female attitudes, with black women considerably more open to accepting gay men as close friends and showing less bias toward homosexuals in general. When we look closer, we also see that African Americans tend to be more conservative in their religious beliefs—a characteristic that relates to homonegativity among white Americans. Black men tend to hold more traditional views about gender roles, another trait that predicts homonegativity among whites, both female and male. African Americans also tend to be disproportionately less well educated and of lower socioeconomic status as a result of the bias they have lived through, and both of these characteristics are related to greater homosexual prejudice for people of all races and ethnicities. Is race the determining factor, or is it a composite of gender, religious views, and educational and income levels?

If A and B happen at the same time (race equals less acceptance of homosexuality), that doesn't mean that A caused B or that B caused A. There could be a C (socioeconomic status) or a D (education) floating out there that may be the real culprit.

The most fascinating of the predictors of negative attitudes toward homosexuality is self-doubt about one's own sexual orientation. Men who are insecure in their own sexual identity express some of the most negative opinions about gay men. In one research study among self-declared heterosexual males, the male college students who expressed the highest level of homonegativity were also those who registered the greatest degree of genital arousal or penile blood flow when shown male-on-male pornography.[15] This phenomenon may be a part of the reason that males tend to show more homonegative attitudes than women and that these attitudes are more strongly directed at gay men as opposed to lesbians. It may not be mere coincidence that some of the most vocal religious and political critics of homosexuality have found themselves embroiled in scandals about their own homosexuality. It also makes you wonder about the men who commit hate crimes against gay men.

STEREOTYPING HOMOSEXUALS AND BISEXUALS

We may not like to admit it, but if we are honest with ourselves, almost all of us operate with stereotypes of one sort or another. We see the Chinese student sitting in the classroom and assume he is among the smartest students in the math class, or we see a mom and dad with the two children and assume the mom is more nurturing than the dad, who may be a great guy, but just not up to a mom's standards. In other instances, our stereotypes offer us a much more negative picture of the other. She speaks to us with a certain Southern accent, and her IQ is lowered by 10 points thanks to our bias. He walks in with his pants hanging below his boxer shorts, and depending on the color of his skin, we pretty well have his story figured out. And then there are the instances when we hold both positive and negative stereotypes about the same group at the same time. We meet the Jewish man and immediately recognize him as bright and successful, but we wonder whether he is going to pay the asking price or we're going to get into a haggling match.

These mental pictures that we carry around in our heads and use as a sort of shorthand for cataloging people often impede our ability to see and understand the beauty and the warts of the person standing in front of us. Even when our pictures have some foundation in statistical truth, we will often miss the truth of the individual.

Homosexuals and bisexuals are clearly not immune from being stereotyped or for that matter from using stereotypes in their own thinking. Throughout this book I have intentionally thrown in more than one or two of these stereotypes: gay man as artistically talented, gay man as good shopper, lesbian as naturalist or environmentalist, lesbian as feminist or assertive leader, bisexual as having the best of both worlds. But of course these stereotypes may often be as wrong as they are right.

The stereotype of professional male dancers as homosexual provides us with one example of the sometimes right, sometimes wrong stereotype. To a certain degree this impression is borne out by a survey of male and female professional dancers who estimate about 58 percent of the men in this profession are gay, a rate higher than would be expected based on overall prevalence figures for homosexuality.[16] Yes, a lot of male dancers are gay, but an estimated 42 percent aren't—these 42 percent think this gives them a wonderful advantage in scoring with some beautiful ballerinas and female dance devotees. Yes, there are straight men who can dance, and anyone who has ever gone dancing with me—straight or gay, male or female—will attest that not all gay men can. What do we know? If he dances on stage, he might be gay, or he could be straight; the odds are 58 to 42 percent. If he is gay, he seems to have a higher probability of being able to dance, but it's not likely he will be the next star of the Alvin Ailey Company. We know enough to know about the group, but not nearly enough to make a judgment about an individual within the group.

In building our first images of homosexuality, we often start with a focus on gender-discordant behaviors that differ from the cultural norm (e.g. the "effeminate" male or overly "butch" female). In turn, these behaviors become our shorthand for homosexuality, with associated terms (e.g., fag or dyke) used as labels of derogation. As with many biases, the stereotypes reflect our discomfort with difference, leading us to label these differences as wrong and even threatening.[17]

Our characterizations of homosexuals take on even greater negative connotations when we hear about gays or lesbians engaging in behaviors that threaten social structures or actions we consider social taboos. These threats may come from nothing more than a challenge to current social mores (e.g., a call for an end to gender bias or misogyny), or the threats may originate from repugnant and criminal behavior (e.g., the child-abuse cases among Catholic priests). And if we are blind to all of the other contributions of LGB persons, these negative images may become our total reality. Ironically, when someone calls our attention to the achievements of homosexuals and bisexuals, we may ask why it is necessary to mention the sexual orientation of heroes and icons—after all, don't questions about Florence Nightingale or Susan B. Anthony's sexual orientation risk taking away from their stature and diminish the work they accomplished? We assume that sexual orientation is something to hide and that it had no impact on the individual's contributions to society, assumptions that exacerbate and reinforce the negative stereotype. (For further discussion, see chapter 9, " Out of the School Closet.")

GAY MEN AND LESBIANS AS GENDER DISCORDANT

Challenging our commonly held perceptions doesn't mean denying that the effeminate male and the butch female are real and thriving members of gay and lesbian communities, as are a number of other varying and even conflicting stereotypes (the hyper-masculine leather man and lipstick lesbian). Instead, in examining these perspectives, we raise questions about whether these highly visible representatives constitute the majority or merely the most often recognized members of the homosexual community. And we question why these characteristics bring about fear or derision.

The fact that drag queens or Dykes on Bikes become symbols of homosexuality is not all that surprising. As some of the more colorful members of the community and, at least at one point, the most willing to be publicly identified, these men and women have frequently been given the largest amount of airtime when the media cover Gay Pride parades or other public rallies. But despite their visibility, it's unlikely that they are the majority or even a large minority of the total gay and lesbian community.[18]

As the gay men and lesbians among us who are members of these cohorts led the parades, many of the rest of us who are less visible remained in the back of the parade or on the sidelines, fearing retribution at work or conflicts with friends and family should we become publicly identified. It's unfortunate that the most colorful members of the gay and lesbian community have, at times, been the only spokespersons for our community as a whole. But even more disappointing is that the members of the gay and lesbian community who stood on the sidelines express embarrassment by the attention paid to our somewhat more theatrical brothers and sisters, an embarrassment that I confess I have felt—an embarrassment borne of my own insecurities.[19]

The phenomenon of calling public attention to the most colorful and, at times, more controversial characters is not unique to media coverage of Gay Pride parades. When television cameras pan football stadiums, more airtime is given to the men and women with foam rubber cheese blocks on their heads than the father and son dressed in the hooded L. L. Bean parkas. Likewise, shots of college students on spring break are more likely to focus on inebriated coeds running around topless than any other group. But even with this media attention, the general public doesn't draw the conclusion that all football fans walk around throughout their daily lives with ridiculous looking hats on their heads and painted skin or that all 19-year-old women are on Florida's beaches taking their tops off.

When those of us who are "mainstream" homosexuals bemoan the fact that our more readily recognized brothers and sisters have become the public image of gay America, we are discounting the contributions that these men and women have made in securing whatever levels of civil protection we currently enjoy. And even worse, we are engaging in our own acts of derision and discrimination. These complaints on our part may be our own internalized homophobia speaking—self-doubt developed over years of hiding from society. The fact that mainstream members of the lesbian and gay community engage in putting someone else down because of her or his differences seems blasphemously hypocritical. It also strengthens the argument that differences can be judged inherently negative.

It is also unfortunate that those of us who are heterosexual hold images of homosexuality drawn from the seemingly outlandish and gender-discordant behaviors of gay men and lesbians. Using these somewhat myopic filters, many of us fail to recognize the full range of behaviors and traits found within the homosexual community. We remain blind to the wonderfully ordinary school teacher, the gay athlete, the war hero, and the lesbian model, reinforcing the idea that these less visible representatives who conform to gender expectations must also remain in the closet if they are to be accepted.

The lack of tolerance for the effeminate male and, to a somewhat lesser degree, intolerance for the masculine female are more a function of societal attitudes about gender roles assumed by heterosexuals than they are about attitudes toward homosexuality. These negative stereotypes of gay men and lesbians reflect and help perpetuate the attitude that there is something wrong or even evil with atypical gender expression. To be valued, all little boys must be on the little league team, and to be loved, little girls should at least sometimes want to wear the party dress—after all, these are their natural given inclinations. It is demeaning for a male to be soft, passive, or effeminate, and it's inappropriate and off-putting for a woman to be assertive and masculine.

GAY MALE AS SEXUALLY WANTON

Although gender-discordant behaviors may be the most common stereotype of the gay male and lesbian, the real and assumed sexual practices of the gay male are often the more damning of our negative images. In many of our minds, gay men are engaged in an unending journey from one sexual orgy to another, and numbers of them are prowling the streets looking for underage boys. These sensationalized renderings are used to raise our greatest fears about same-sex behaviors.

The body of evidence certainly does point to differences in the sexual practices of homosexual and heterosexual men, with gay men having more sexual partners. But to fully appreciate what these data tell us, we have to look at several variables at the same time. Cross-cultural studies indicate that in addition to our sexual orientation, our gender and marital status, as well as other social influences, are related to differences in our sexual behaviors and sexual attitudes.[20]

As indicated by this research, those of us who are homosexual men report having more sexual partners than do those of us who are heterosexual men. At the same time, those of us who are men—straight or gay—report having greater numbers of sexual partners than do those of us who are female. As men, regardless of our sexual orientation, we also report thinking about having sex more frequently in the course of the day than do women, although these differences certainly don't indicate asexuality on the part of women. In addition, straight and gay men show more liberal attitudes about our sexual practices (e.g., less concern with fidelity, more willingness to have casual sex, and more interest in having sex with multiple partners at one time).

Would heterosexual men have more sexual partners if women were equally interested in having sex? Reports on the sex lives of rock stars and professional male athletes suggest that the answer is yes. Probably the most staggering number from this group is Wilt Chamberlin's quite possibly exaggerated claim to have had sex with some 20,000 women (Swift 1992).

When we look at differences among women, we find that those of us who are heterosexual and homosexual women look similar in terms of both attitudes and behavior, whereas bisexual women report more liberal attitudes and sexual behavior patterns. But all three of these groups fall below homosexual and heterosexual male norms for the number of sexual partners and for liberal or promiscuous attitudes.[21]

Not surprisingly, regardless of gender, those of us who are unmarried report having more partners than our married peers; however, those of us who are married men and women report having sex more frequently than our unmarried counterparts.[22] We may have fewer partners, but if we are married or in a committed relationship, our one partner is in bed with us every night and on weekend afternoons. The relatively newly married heterosexual couple who lived in the apartment next to mine several years ago had a more active sex life than I have ever had; I confess I was jealous.

In addition to differences based on gender and sexual orientation, the number of sexual partners we have also varies based on our geographic location, our educational level, and our social and religious views.[23] If we are college educated, we report having more partners than if we are high school graduates. And if we have more liberal social and religious views, we report having more partners than if we are more conservative in our values. If we are male and living in a major metropolitan area, we are also likely to have more partners than if we are male but living in a rural area.

When we examine all of these data, we realize that multiple factors may account for the differences in our sexual behaviors, including our sexual orientation. If we are a homosexual male, we are likely to have more sexual partners than if we are a heterosexual male. One possible explanation for the difference in the numbers is an artifact of the male of the species being more open to having sexual relations than his female peers, making it easier for those of us who are homosexual males to find greater numbers of sexual partners, given that our target is typically another man who is also open to having sexual relationships. A part of the difference may also be attributable to an increased emphasis on and even social reward for promiscuous behavior within gay culture. If you are a gay male, you gain status by having more partners, proving you are more desirable. If you are a heterosexual male, your male peers may give you bonus points, but the women you are seeking to date may not bestow the same honor on you. Your ratings may actually decline in their eyes if you have too many partners. The fact that bisexual women report different behavior patterns than their heterosexual and homosexual peers also may be attributed to greater opportunity (i.e., being open to having sex with men and women) and to their more liberal attitudes. Another part of the explanation may rest in the fact that: if you are a gay male you are more likely to relocate to a major metropolitan area, seeking a more open and accepting social network. If you are a lesbian, you are less likely to relocate.

These discussions bring us back to society's nature-versus-nurture discussions. If males, straight and gay, are inherently inclined to spread their seed because of an evolutionary advantage, it might be expected that men seek more partners than women and that gay men not only seek but also find greater numbers of sexual partners, despite the fact that they are not engaged in procreation.[24] On the other hand, if men, both heterosexual and homosexual, are socialized to concentrate on sex more and to value casual sex over fidelity, we could also anticipate homosexual men to seek more partners than their female counterparts and to find more willing partners than their straight male peers.[25] Either of these hypotheses would be strengthened by the fact that gay men's lives are not governed by social forces that act as controls on heterosexual men's behavior (e.g., the expectation of socially sanctioned marriage and fidelity, the influence of conservative religious doctrine).

Unfortunately, facts that would help to deepen our knowledge of the sexual practices of homosexual, bisexual, and heterosexual men and women are not available in the data we have to date. For example, some commentaries suggest that long-term relationships, especially when openly acknowledged and supported by family and social networks, may mitigate the number of partners,[26] but we are only beginning to collect the data to examine these assumptions. If these commentaries prove to be true, we could postulate that providing access to state-sanctioned marriage could alter sexual practices among gay men. I certainly have a number of friends who live in committed relationships that suggest this may be true; two of the dearest just celebrated their 55th anniversary, and Will and Mac, two other friends, hit 35 years this year. Another of the findings that we can't explain with current data is the significant variance in the number of partners among gay men, with most falling far short of the numbers that make the sensationalized headlines.

Examining the research that we have available, it seems reasonable to assume that gender is one of two overriding variables in determining the number of partners, with sexual orientation as practiced in today's culture being the other. As discussed previously, it is possible that these gender differences could be attributable to nature or nurture. Personally, I am betting on nature, with nurture and society blended in. Homosexual men probably don't think about sex any more often than our heterosexual brothers might, but when we are in a bar, we have a greater likelihood of scoring because we are talking to other men who are also spending a lot of time thinking about sex. Plus, we don't have any rules set up by a government or church-sanctioned marriage. If we are a heterosexual man in the bar, we are targeting women who may very well have a different view on sex.

GAY MALE AS PEDOPHILE

Voices from our church and political pulpits use the number of sexual partners as a springboard in building the stereotype of gay man as pedophile and child abuser: "These men are not only having sex with more people; they want to have sex with our young sons"—a frightening thought for any parent. With the painfully real reports of Catholic priests abusing children in parishes across America (and the globe, for that matter), along with the echoes of demands to lower the age of consensual sex coming from a dying organization named NAMBLA (North American Man/Boy Love Association) and occasional commentaries by queer theorists, we may wonder if there is truth in this stereotype of the gay man as a predator seeking out children and adolescents. (See chapter 8 in this text for a discussion on NAMBLA.)

One way we can begin understanding this stereotype is to look at our own reactions to those who are different from us under somewhat less dramatic circumstances. When we see someone as being different, there is an increased likelihood that we will attribute bothersome or offensive behaviors to those differences. Allow me to propose one such example, recognizing that you may have a better one for yourself.

When the driver next to us cuts us off, if the driver is like us—same gender, same age, same race—he or she is an individual idiot. But when the driver is of a different gender, age, or race/ethnicity, she or he becomes a "typical woman," a "testosterone Tony," a "senile old man," or a "crazy (fill in the ethnic slur)." In reporting on sex crimes, we can track a similar reaction. If it is a case of male-on-male child abuse, sexual orientation is likely to become a focus of attention, suggesting a link between homosexuality and child abuse. However, when the heterosexual male commits a similar crime against a young girl, sexual orientation goes without comment. The horror of the crime remains the focus, with us looking for other answers to the question of why. Although it's not one of our better or nobler characteristics, distrust of the other may be one of those traits that we will need to fight against as we evolve as a species. (See the section on Sodom and Gomorrah in chapter 4 for further discussion on this topic.)

In considering the stereotype of gay male as pedophile, we need to look closely and thoroughly at the numbers. When we examine the numbers, the first thing we see is that there are significantly more male-on-female sexual abuse cases with children than there are incidents of male-on-male abuse.[27] At the same time, we find that the percent of reported cases of male-on-male sexual abuse is higher than estimated rates of homosexuality in the male population. In various research studies, male-on-male child abuse cases account for 9 to 40 percent of the total number of reported crimes, which is higher than our 6 percent estimate for the number of gay males in the population.

If these figures are accurate, aren't the critics of gay rights correct—gay men are more likely to commit sexual abuse than heterosexual man? For at least two different reasons, we need to be careful about interpreting these numbers quite so quickly.[28] First, we need to consider the fact that most male-on-male child abuse occurs outside of the family, whereas young girls have a higher likelihood of being victims of incestuous abuse. Knowing this, it's important to understand that sex crimes that occur outside the family are more likely to be reported than are sex crimes that occur within the family structure, where they are often hidden. If your son is attacked by a neighbor, stranger, or family friend, you are going to call the police. If your daughter is attacked by an uncle or grandfather, as angry as you are, you still may take a different course of action, forbidding the uncle or grandfather from being alone with or ever seeing your little girl again. You want the neighbor or stranger prosecuted, but you don't want to see the relative in jail; you just want your child protected from further abuse. This means that when we examine data on child abuse, we see only a small fraction of the cases of incest (crimes involving little girls being attacked by family members) but a much larger percentage of the cases committed by men from outside the home (the types of crimes where little boys are attacked).

The next fact we need to consider is that many of the men who attack little boys are heterosexual in their adult sex lives. Pedophilia (repeated attacks against prepubescent children) and hebophilia (repeated attacks against teenagers) are not acts of sexual attraction or love, and the men who engage in them may have different adult sexual relationships than their crimes would indicate. In one study, Jenny and his fellow researchers examined 269 cases of sexual abuse with children where the perpetrator was an adult. In 50 (or 18.5%) of the cases, the victim was a male child. In 37 of these 50 cases (74%), the perpetrator was or had been in a heterosexual relationship with the child's mother, foster mother, grandmother, or other female relative. Three of the boys were attacked by adult women, and one was attacked by his mother and father. Only 4 (or 1.5%) of the 269 child abuse cases were male-on-male attacks committed by men who were living their adult sex lives as homosexuals. Although intuition may tell us that a man who attacks a little boy probably is homosexual, the data suggest this is not always true. We need much more detailed data to make a clear determination on this.

So what do we know about the stereotype? We know that men are more likely to commit sexual abuse on children than are women. We know that the data tell us that little girls are more vulnerable to these attacks than are boys. And we strongly believe that there is a greater underreporting of attacks on little girls because these attacks are often incestuous in nature and thus hidden from public records. We also know that when little boys are attacked, it is more often a non–family member who perpetrates the crime, and often the male perpetrators are heterosexual in their adult sex lives. And thankfully, we know that the vast majority of men, heterosexual and homosexual, don't engage in these terrible crimes. We also know that linking child sex abuse to homosexuality is a great scare tactic, which can cause a believer to question the wisdom of the homosexual teacher, pediatrician, cleric, or child care worker.[29]

LESBIAN AS "FEMINAZI"

Although gay men may be seen by some of us as a threat to our sons or grandsons' safety, lesbians and their feminist agendas are at times viewed as a threat to our social order. Certainly, Americans have long come to closure on first-wave feminist issues: Yes, women in the United States and around the world should have the right to vote, they are not their husbands' property, and they should be educated. We have also adopted, if not completely accepted, most but not all of the initiatives that came out of the second wave of feminist ideas: equal pay is the right way to go, female athletes should be given the same chance in school as male athletes, and reproductive rights are part of our law, if not fully accepted. But the Equal Rights Amendment never did get approved.[30]

Conservative talk show host Rush Limbaugh is credited with introducing the derogatory term *feminazi* into the public conversation. The term is a contraction or compounding of *feminist* and *Nazi.*

There has been a price to pay in getting society to this point on feminist issues, and there continue to be political costs for maintaining the status quo. Taking the movement further seems to be getting harder and continues to result in some interesting battles, inside and outside the feminist tent.

At the same time that feminists can thank lesbian activists for some of the movement's greatest successes, there are some who feel that visible and vocal lesbian involvement has caused significant distraction in the struggle. Some lesbian activists have, in turn, claimed that the only way to be a true feminist is to be a lesbian-feminist. And the loudest critics of feminism have recognized that if they can conflate the various issues, then all they need to do to get many of the rest of us to show disdain for everyone under the tent is to get us to disagree on two or three hot-button issues—reproductive rights, whether women should be on the frontline in war, and whether being a mom really has to be tied to being a wife.

Lesbians and bisexual women have played an important role throughout the history of feminism, beginning with the women's suffrage movement. But in their early roles, their sexual orientation was rarely if ever acknowledged and never a key element of the debates. These were women fighting for the rights of women, not lesbians or bisexuals fighting for the rights of women. That changed in the 1970s, as more and more out and vocal lesbians and bisexual women began to walk away from the gay liberation movement and join their straight sisters in the women's movement. As this occurred, opponents of feminism started to level claims that the women's movement was being hijacked by lesbians. Heterosexual feminists became uncomfortable with the Lavender Menace and worked to take the spotlight off lesbian involvement. This created one of the several fractures in the feminist movement, with some high-profile lesbians starting splinter organizations while they asserted that the only way for women to truly come into their own was to separate from men, and the only true feminists were lesbian-feminists, allowing for political lesbians (i.e., heterosexual women who gave up having sex with men).[31]

Now all of this became very confusing—who was a lesbian, and who was a political lesbian; who was a feminist, and who wasn't? These discussions opened up attacks and counterattacks from inside and outside the tent. Heterosexual feminists were traitors to womanhood and had capitulated with heterosexism. Lesbian feminists were insisting that their agenda become everywoman's agenda and threatening all the progress the women's movement had made to date. It was clear that feminism had accomplished some good things (the vote, equal pay), but now it was threatening men, heterosexuality, and the family and society in general. Everyone had an enemy and a complaint.

So where are we today, and are the stereotypes true? Are all lesbians feminists, are all feminists lesbians, and would all lesbians and all feminists prefer men to disappear from the face of the earth? The simple answer is there is no *all,* but there certainly are *some.* No, not all feminists are lesbians. Most, but by no means all, lesbians consider themselves to be feminists.[32] And their various definitions of what it means to be a feminist range far and wide. Some are concerned with economic and legal constraints on women; some focus on opening all of society to feminist values of caring, peace, and respect for ecology; some say we must focus on the oppression of race at the same time we focus on women's issues; and some support and bring to life the idea of women-only communities. How many fit into each category? We don't have the data to answer this question. Dawn Szymanski's study does suggest that 74 percent of lesbians and bisexual women identify themselves as feminists, 10 percent disavow the label of feminist, and 16 percent are sitting on the fence. My experience tells me that very few lesbians fit into the let's-live-separated-from-men category. Of course, I wouldn't be likely to run into those that did fit this label very often, would I? I did, however, live not far from one such community, just as I have lived close to gated and retirement communities. I have never been threatened personally by any of these communities.

LESBIANS AS BUTCH AND FEMME COUPLES

Growing up in a conservative Protestant household, I remember a period when as a child I was fascinated by the nuns in habits I would occasionally see walking in our neighborhood. They were teachers at the neighborhood Catholic school. I created various childhood theories about these women in black. It seemed to me that they were always in pairs of twos and that one would be tall and one would be short or one would be thin and one would be overweight. When I was in my twenties, and the habits had disappeared, I shared some of my observations with Sister Mary Francis, a dear sainted friend who had been in an order when the habit was still worn; she suggested that my theories were wrong and most likely predicated on a fascination with the exotic and the rare. I suspect that some of our ideas about lesbian couples may be based on the same fascination with what we may see as the mysterious.

A week ago, as I was doing the mandatory Saturday grocery shopping, I ran across a lesbian couple that I often see at the local supermarket. I am not sure if they had come shopping after some particular event, but they were proudly celebrating their relationship by the outfits they were wearing that afternoon—matching shorts and shirts—much like the occasional mother–daughter, twin sister, or even more rare husband–wife teams we run across. As clearly as their wardrobe said "we belong together," their hairstyles (one long and curled and one short and spiked), their differing mannerisms (one gave me a big smile and wave, whereas the other was much more reserved), and their differing body types declared them a wonderful and happy example of the butch-femme stereotype.

The following night I was having dinner at two friends' house. On the guest list were two of Mac and Will's closest friends and travel buddies, Nan and Dianne. In this relationship, if you tried to pick out who was butch and who was femme, you would have to base your decision on which one was wearing the least amount of lipstick that evening. Of course, if you ran into them on another evening at a concert in the city, you might have to re-order your thoughts about who was butch and who was femme based on who was wearing the silver lemay scarf around her neck and who was wearing the solid black scarf draped over one shoulder. These two women defy definition based on the butch–femme dichotomy.

And then there is Jen and Sammie, the two women who took me under their wings when I was in my late teens; both seemed pretty butch to me, especially when they would take me to target practice. And both seemed very motherly as they tried to help me navigate through part of my coming-out process.

Although there are lesbian couples who have clear role differentiation in their public personas, there are many who don't. It also should be no surprise that in any one of these relationships, what you see in public may or may not be what you find when it comes to the division of labor around the house—"you clean the house, and I'll do the home repairs" versus "you clean the house, and I'll do the laundry and grocery shopping," or "I'll do the plumbing; you take care of the lawn." And when it comes to what happens in each couple's respective bedrooms, I have to leave that to someone else to discuss. This may be the only place where I apply a personal I-don't-ask-and-please-don't-tell policy. I will leave that to the couples themselves and to their male heterosexual neighbors who may or may not be fantasizing.

In thinking about these three couples, what does seem to be happening is that each couple has challenged one or another of the premises offered not only by general society but also by the various schools of lesbian feminism or queer theory. In some eyes, my grocery-shopping buddies have bought into a patriarchal-heterosexist model, my lipstick-wearing dinner companions are conforming to the *Vogue* model of womanhood, and my target-practice mentors were aping father values along with those of mother. These couples are attacked from outside and from inside the community. But then, I find it disconcerting when I hear my heterosexual friends describe what's wrong in the way their neighbors are organizing their heterosexual families—she works outside the home and has abandoned her children; she stays home and doesn't contribute anything to their household income, and now they can't afford to clothe their children; he comes home and sits in front of the television while she waits on him; she makes him do everything—she is such a princess. I know there are wrong ways to structure any given relationship—you don't beat up your spouse or partner, for example—but I suspect there are multiple right ways to express love and build family. In all three cases of the lesbians I have mentioned here, it seems to me that they are happy and contributing members of society, so I for one am willing to let them lead their lives in the structure they find most comfortable.

LESBIANS AND GAY MEN AS EMOTIONALLY DISTURBED AND UNSTABLE

After pointing to gender-discordant behaviors, sexual promiscuity, and what some would call radical social movements, if you wanted to continue raising objections to society's growing acceptance of LGB individuals, you could try to draw connections between homosexuality and emotional or behavioral disorders: "Recent studies show that homosexuals have a substantially greater risk of suffering from a psychiatric problem than do heterosexuals."[33] Asserting that gay men, lesbians, or bisexuals are inherently emotionally disturbed and that these disorders show up in depression, suicidal tendencies, and domestic partner abuse sets the stage for yet one more reason to cure or rid ourselves and our society of homosexuality. When we cure homosexuality, we will eliminate the behavioral and emotional disorders.

Thinking back to our example of the bad driver who is the same as us ("that idiot") versus the bad driver who is different from us ("that senile old man," etc.), if we are a heterosexual male, what goes through our minds when we hear about a neighbor who beats up his wife? We are probably distressed by his behavior and attribute it to some individual characteristic deep within him, but we don't see it as being part of the typical male psyche. Now, what do we think when we hear about a lesbian the next block over abusing her partner? If we have a lesbian sister with whom we are close, we probably pray that never happens to her just as we hope our daughter never has to face the treatment our neighbor inflicted on his wife. If, on the other hand, we oppose homosexual and bisexual rights, we may see this as one more reason not to give gays or lesbians the right to marriage. Doesn't the lesbian attacking her partner provide us with one more piece of evidence that homosexuals are emotionally unstable and unfit for marriage?

If you are a heterosexual reading this text, let me share a little secret—my LGB brothers and sisters and I are human. Some of us are wonderfully grounded, and some of us are, quite frankly, terribly screwed up in the head, as is our heterosexual neighbor who beats his wife. Whether hetero- or homo- or bisexual, we come in all sizes, shapes, colors, and forms. And this means that there is domestic partner abuse in both gay and straight relationships, something that wasn't really recognized until the 1990s.[34] What the emerging data indicate is that the alarmingly high rates of abuse we see in heterosexual relationships are mirrored in same-sex couples, both male and female, with physical violence and verbal or psychological abuse occurring in as many as one-fourth of all households.[35]

When we think of heterosexual relationships and domestic violence, most of us have an image of the power imbalance between men and women. But how do we frame this abuse in same-gender relationships? Some of our conservative pundits offer the "inherent mental instability of the homosexual" as the root of the problem. On the other hand, the research tells us that within same-sex relationships, we see the same unfortunate demons we find in heterosexual relationships: power imbalance, substance abuse, repeating patterns of abuse seen in childhood, jealousy, and dependency, and these demons can be exacerbated by internalized homonegativity or homophobia.[36] Those gay men and lesbians who show higher degrees of negative feelings about self and about homosexuality are less likely to have successful relationships.

If we are bothered by domestic abuse in the LGB community, the answer isn't to nurture the negative self-image—"If you could overcome your homosexuality, you wouldn't abuse your partner or allow yourself to be abused." If we care about the victim and the perpetrator, we need to help them learn to accept themselves—one of the most important of the several steps to wholeness. In contrast to the would-be therapeutic approaches such as Exodus and other ex-gay ministries, the therapy needed in these situations helps resolve the negative self-image. (See chapter 5 on the "ex-gay" identity and ministry.)

Just as domestic violence is a serious problem for adults in relationships, suicide is a tragedy that affects all too many teenagers. But unlike the domestic violence data, the data on adolescent suicide tell us this is especially true for LGBT youth.[37] In studies examining this phenomenon, researchers have found increased probability of suicide related to gender-nonconforming behavior, parental rejection, and social disapproval, with the effects of gender-nonconforming behaviors being significantly more apparent among gay boys than lesbians.[38] If you are an LGBT youth, you have a greater likelihood of experiencing suicidal thoughts, engaging in suicidal attempts, and committing suicide. But if we can build an environment in which you are accepted at home and in the neighborhood, we can decrease the risk of your committing suicide and increase your well-being.[39]

A neighbor of one of our staff members recently confided in Brigitte that the neighbor suspected her son might be gay. When Brigitte asked the neighbor how she felt about that, the woman said that if Ian was gay, she knew he would burn in Hell.

This is not an atypical initial, and in some cases lifelong, response for parents who discover their children are homosexual. Regrettably, as these parents work through their own emotional reactions, they are likely to be damaging their children's mental well-being.

Recognizing the suicide rates among LGBT youth, those of us who are homosexual rights advocates have asked schools to address this problem by providing support services for these students. More recently and as a counterargument, those who oppose LGBT rights have suggested that the higher suicide rate among LGBT youth means we need to find ways to cure homosexuality—if we can change homosexuality into heterosexuality, we will lessen the risk of suicide. The problem with this speculation is that if suicide is not a direct result of being homosexual, but is rather the result of self-doubt and self-hatred spawned by societal rejection, then attempts to cure homosexuality will most likely cause more self-hatred, making the problem even worse. As Mom and Dad are praying for Chris to be healed of homosexuality, Chris is aware of Mom and Dad's rejection, and the risk of suicide and other mental health problems looms even larger.

As in the case of domestic violence and teenage suicides, we have several questions we need to ask ourselves before we draw conclusions about the relationships between emotional and behavioral problems and the individual's sexual orientation. Our first question needs to be whether we see the same incidence rates of a particular mental health issue in the LGB population as in the general population. If the answer is the same or close to the same, as is the case with domestic violence, that's what we would expect. Where we find higher rates among homosexuals and bisexuals, as with teen suicide, we need to ask a second question: is the behavior or emotional disorder the result of being homosexual, or is it the result of being shunned, isolated, berated, or punished for being different—that is, for being homosexual? If the answer is the latter, the solution can't be found in converting the individual to heterosexuality, which may well be impossible. (See chapter 5, "Reparative Therapy and the Ex-Gay Identity.") The immediate answer rests in equipping the individual to cope with and develop resilience in the face of these negative messages. Fortunately, most LGB individuals find mechanisms to accomplish this on their own. The long-range answer is to build a more accepting society. We are on the road to doing this, but there are a number of obstacles and bumps in the road ahead.

LESBIANS AND GAY MEN AS LIBERAL VOICES

I have on more than one occasion imposed on a friend who was a remarkably successful Republican big-city mayor, turned even more successful university president, to serve as the guest of honor at fundraisers for two different organizations that serve the needs of LGBT youth. John has graciously accepted and been a big draw. Each time he has accepted, he has reminded me that he doubts that many of the people in the room would have voted for him. In joking around about it, I tell him that in his second election he ran unopposed, so he got some of my tribe's votes, and that he has great-looking hair, so I am sure he got some gay votes in that first election too. But despite John's individual popularity across demographics, a Hunter College poll suggests that in most political campaigns he is correct: out gays and lesbians are much more likely to vote Democrat.[40] But what causes that to be true, and what about those gays and lesbians who are still in the closet?

Dee Mosbacher, a well-recognized psychiatrist, is also daughter of Robert Mosbacher, a former cabinet member and director of George W. Bush's second campaign for the White House. Although the family is supportive of Dee and her partner, there have been times when the political differences between father and daughter have been highlighted in the news.

When Dee and her father were delivering commencement addresses to two different colleges on the same day, Dee began hers by saying: "Dad and I had breakfast this morning. We had a look at each other's speeches. He would have used mine, but he is not a lesbian. I would have used his, but I am not a Republican" (Bernstein 2003, 171).

Although we know that there are homosexual and bisexual conservatives, national polls do indicate that the majority of self-identified bisexuals, lesbians, and gay men tend to express more liberal attitudes with regard to politics and religion.[41] This isn't particularly surprising, but it does raise the cause-effect questions we talked about earlier in this chapter.

There is certainly no basis for believing that homosexuals are more likely to be born into liberal homes. Consider Mary Cheney, daughter of former vice president Dick Cheney; John Schlafly, son of Phyllis Schlafly, the founder of the Eagle Forum, a conservative women's group; Ty Ross, Barry Goldwater's grandson; and Candace Gingrich, half-sister of former conservative Speaker of the House Newt Gingrich—each of these individuals provides high-profile evidence of this. So is it life experience that makes bisexuals, gay men, and lesbians liberal?

In many ways former Wisconsin Congressman Steve Gunderson's story is similar to that of long time Massachusetts Congressman Barney Frank. Both were elected to Congress after serving in their state legislatures, both were seen as bright and articulate members of the House. And both came out as being gay when the press pushed the issue. A Democrat, Frank continues to serve successfully years after coming out. A Republican, Gunderson was encouraged by party officials not to run for reelection after he came out, even though the seat went to a Democrat when Gunderson stepped aside (Gunderson and Morris 1996).

Questions about gays and lesbians being born to liberal parents or becoming more liberal as a result of life experiences could be the wrong questions. The data could be telling us that those of us who are homosexual and hold more liberal views find it easier to acknowledge and detail our sexual orientation on surveys than our homosexual sisters and brothers who view the world in more conservative terms. What might be happening is that conservative homosexuals are skewing the results of our surveys by their unwillingness or inability to answer the questions about their sexual orientation openly and honestly. Their conservative attitudes may force them to stay closeted on surveys of sexual attraction and behavior and even more so on surveys of self-identity. Thus, these conservative-leaning homosexuals and bisexuals go uncounted in our prevalence estimates. And this means we have no solid data on how many homosexuals there are and in particular how many conservative homosexuals there are. We have seen some highly publicized outings among conservative politicians and evangelical clergy, and more likely than not, these men denied their sexual orientation on any anonymous surveys they may have taken before and even after these outings: "Are you homosexual?" No. "Did you vote Democrat?" No. "Did you vote Republican?" Yes.

In considering the question of whether homosexuals have more liberal values, as the national polls would indicate, we might also ask if the very process of coming out forces the individual to adopt more liberal attitudes as suggested by the study from Hunter College and the Human Rights Commission.[42] Or it could be that coming out draws the individual to associate with people who are more liberal in their ideas, influencing the LGB indi-

> Johann Hari, a columnist for the *London Independent,* provides some very disturbing facts for those of us who would like to believe that being gay should inoculate us from neoconservative views. In a 2008 blog posting, Hari outed a set of neo-fascist leaders in Europe as being homosexual. Several of these men had previously admitted that they were gay (Hari 2008).
>
> You have to wonder how someone could live in Germany or Austria and miss the point of what Hitler did to the gay and lesbian community during his reign of terror.

vidual's worldviews. Among my friends, those who are the most conservative tend to be the most closeted, and those who are the most open tend to be the most liberal in their general political beliefs. But as always, this is not an absolute.

What we can say about this characterization is that openly gay men, lesbians, and bisexuals are more likely to be liberal. But there are gays and lesbians who are out of the closet and who hold conservative values and vote accordingly. And there are major disputes between the two groups. What we don't know is whether closeted homosexuals and bisexuals are more conservative and how many of them there are.

CREATING A NEW STEREOTYPE—THE LESBIAN/GAY PARENT AS ???

We have seen a number of shifts in the character and structure of the American family throughout the 20th century and going into the 21st, with recent data showing an increase in the percent of children being raised by two homosexual-parent households as well as an increase in the percentage of children being raised in cohabitating households and in children living without parents. At the same time, there has been a decline in the percent of children being raised by single mothers and in particular by nonworking single mothers.[43] Another part of this changing landscape of the American family has been a growth in the number of children being raised in households with two same-sex birth/adoptive/foster parents at the helm.

In many of the instances with households headed by same-sex partners, we are asking family court judges to make decisions premised on strikingly different portrayals of lesbians and gay males as parents and on opposing characterizations of the health of households headed by same-sex couples. In one set of pictures, we portray same-sex households as hotbeds of contagion where children are being deprived of dual-gender parenting and exposed to and encouraged to adopt homosexuality as a way of life.[44] The parents in these households are cast as male pedophiles and man-hating lesbians who endanger the lives of the children placed in their homes. The attorneys representing these women and men in adoption and custody cases are countering these assertions with a very different picture. In their arguments before the court, these advocates are pointing to research that shows lesbian and gay couples raising heterosexual children in homes that look much the same as the homes headed by opposite-sex couples. The children raised in these homes grow up to have the same level of self-esteem and psychological well-being as their peers who grew up with heterosexual parents. In the cases where there are differences, at least some of the differences favor the child raised by same-sex parents—same-sex couples who adopt are more financially stable than the average heterosexual couples that adopt, gay fathers are more attentive parents than heterosexual fathers, and lesbian mothers are raising sons who are less aggressive and pay more attention in school.[45]

So which of these dueling stereotypes better reflects the truth? Stacey and Biblarz present a strong argument that both pictures are flawed, but to very different degrees.[46] Of necessity, much of the research we conduct to determine whether there are differences in children raised in households headed by same-sex parents compared to children raised in other types of households—single mother, stepparents, two birth parents, adoptive parents—have used nonrandom samples. This is a common weakness in much of our research on humans and limits how far we can generalize the results. This problem is further exacerbated by the fact that much of this research has been limited to middle-class, predominantly white families. When we see similar results in several different studies, it helps us allay our fears about using nonrandom samples; replicating a nonrandom study with other samples helps build some comfort level. But the only way we are going to know how things work in non-middle-class and non-white families is to study these groups directly. Different cultural norms probably mean differences in parenting patterns in households headed by homosexual and heterosexual parents.

Another of the problems with some of the earlier research, which is being corrected today, is the failure to examine some inconvenient details that may arise in the results. For example, although children raised in households headed by same-sex parents do fare well on a number of measures, these children do appear to be subject to greater social stigma.[47] This increased stigma is not surprising; children of mixed-race marriages have experienced and continue to experience similar stigma. But we wouldn't consider stopping such marriages or family arrangements based on this. Instead we hope that society will eventually grow up, and it slowly but surely is doing so. After all, we have elected a president of the United States who was the product of such a household, and yes, he has paid a price for his parents' atypical marriage, but I think he has shown that you can survive the pettiness exhibited by some elements of society and in spite or because of it make something of yourself.

The data that we have used in courts and state legislatures to oppose homosexual adoption have as often as not emanated from the Family Research Institute, an organization headed by a psychologist named Paul Cameron. Cameron has the distinction of being the only psychologist to have been expelled from the American Psychological Association for violations of ethical principles, disassociated from the Nebraska Psychological Association for similar behavior, and publically chastised by the American Sociological Association for misrepresentation of sociological research.[48] Those who oppose adoption by homosexuals often base their claims on Cameron's work, which reputedly shows that children raised by same-sex parents are likely to become inculcated into being homosexual themselves and that little boys raised by gay fathers are likely to be sexually molested by their fathers.[49] If you took the errors we found in Kinsey's, Beiber's, and Spitzer's research combined, you might find the amount of error found in Cameron's original research as well as his reinterpretation of data collected and reported by other researchers. But lest those who support homosexual adoption and other parenting practices crow too loudly, we need to remember that there are some weaknesses in the research we rely on too, although these weaknesses are far from the methodological sins Cameron commits.

On the Saturday morning that I was sitting in a local Starbucks in Jacksonville, Florida, typing these passages, I came across six examples of families that could have posed for a 1950s or 1960s Norman Rockwell magazine cover, except for the fact that in three of the cases, the parents were gay or lesbian. In my first encounter, I struck up a conversation with a young mother who was having her coffee while doting on her four-month-old son, Isaiah, a child who was all smiles. Mom allowed me to hold Isaiah, and that was all I needed to make my day. Then the second mother of the day and a dad walked in with two toddlers, the oldest of whom was after everything he could get his hands on, as any three-year-old should be. His father was trying to keep track of him while his mom held his little sister and placed the family order. The next family to appear on the scene was a dad and a dad, both white, with their six- or seven-year-old African American daughter standing in between them, holding on to her taller father's hand. She was dressed in cute little jeans with pink embroidery on the back pocket, the mandatory pink belt, and—you guessed it—the pink t-shirt. Dad number 2, who wasn't holding his daughter's hand, placed the order for three drinks without consulting his partner or his daughter. Obviously, he knew the drill. The fourth family looked like a younger version of the third, two dads and one daughter, except in this case the daughter was much younger, was white, and was being held by her shorter-statured father. Family 5 was two lesbians and two children, a son who was around 10 years old and a daughter who I estimate to have been 13. By facial features, hair color, and build, the boy had to be the birth son of one of the moms, and the daughter was probably the other mother's birth child. But you couldn't tell these relationships by patterns of interaction. The boy was leaning against his non-biological mother while the girl was engaging in conversation about responsibilities with her non-birth mother. The last family to enter the coffee shop was a dad and his three teenagers, each of them trying to decide what they wanted to drink and each one shouting orders at their dad, who obviously took great pleasure in having his children together.

As I saw these families parade in and out over the course of the hour or so that I was there, I felt wonderful about our future as a human family. In each case all that I saw was unconditional love. Now, I know that you can't make any judgments from five minutes of watching anyone. And yes, I recognized that the numbers were all off—two gay male couples versus one lesbian couple versus three what I assumed to be heterosexual-led households is far from representative of America's family structures, but it certainly was a heartwarming slice of the pie. And it sure beat seeing a mom screaming and yelling at the kid at the grocery store or the dad ignoring the children as mom was trying to hold the family together. My America was beautiful that morning.

STRAIGHT TALK

As with all stereotypes, characterizations about homosexuals and bisexuals should cause us to raise some fairly standard questions, the first of these being, is the stereotype an accurate portrayal, or are we taking a single example or small number of cases and overgeneralizing to the whole?

Reading the story about domestic violence in one lesbian household, do we take this to mean that lesbians are violent, or does it indicate to us that this one woman has serious emotional and behavioral problems that make her unfit to be in a relationship that is supposed to be marked by love—just like the man two blocks over who beats his wife? Do we see the man who sexually abuses young boys as representative of all gay men, or do we see him as we see the man who preys on young girls—a lone, bad actor?

When we find that there is a higher incidence rate for a given characteristic in the gay or lesbian population, our second question should be, are we seeing a behavior or trait that is the result of being homosexual, or is it a trait associated with being lesbian or gay but caused by another set of variables? Do gay men have more sexual partners than their heterosexual peers because homosexuality itself triggers greater sexual appetite or because they are men who are seeking other men minus any social regulator? When we hear of the increased rates of suicide among gay and lesbian teenagers, do we see this as a problem inherent within homosexuals, or do we understand the vulnerability many of us experience in our teenage years and acknowledge the added stress that comes with being a young person who is being rejected by family and society? This question is the same as asking ourselves whether the rate of violence among African American males is the result of an inherited characteristic or whether it results from poverty and other social forces.

A third question we want to ask ourselves is whether the differences we see really matter. If a male is identified as being gay because he is more effeminate, or a female is thought of as a lesbian because she is more masculine, does it really matter? There are certainly gay men and lesbians who are identified as being homosexual because of these traits. But not all lesbians are masculine, and not all butch women are lesbians. The same is true about effeminate men. And quite frankly, what difference does it make? What does it say about us when we find ourselves uncomfortable with an effeminate man or masculine woman? Is that how we judge the value of a person, based on his or her score on a masculinity-versus-femininity scale?

Individual gay men and lesbians do some terrible and frightening things to themselves and others, as do individual heterosexual men and women. But as with our heterosexual peers, LGB men and women also make some remarkable contributions to family, friends, and society at large. Seen or unseen, those of us who are LGB helped settle this country and win its freedom, we added to its literature and its arts, and we are helping to raise and educate its children. We are part of the fabric of this society, as we have been throughout history.

NOTES

1. Santosuosso 2004, 118.
2. Katz 1976, 281–333.
3. Leupp 1995, 205–18.
4. Beck 1999, 56.
5. Saad 2008.
6. Andersen and Fetner 2008.
7. Pew Research Center 2007.
8. Stulhofer and Rimac 2009.
9. N. Sullivan 1995.
10. Walls 2008.
11. Herek 2003b; Walls 2008.
12. Andersen and Fetner 2008.
13. Herek 2003b.
14. Battle and Lemelle 2002; Herek 2003b.
15. Adams, Wright, and Lohr 1996.
16. Bailey and Oberschneider 1997.
17. Fone 2000; Herek 2003b; Simon 1998.
18. Taywaditep 2002.
19. Bawer 1994; Loftin 2007.
20. Laumann, Gagnon, Michael, and Michaels 1994; Johnson, Wadsworth, Wellings and Field 1994; Schmitt 2006.
21. Schmitt 2006.
22. Laumann, Gagnon, Michael and Michaels 1994.
23. Laumann, Gagnon, Michael, and Michaels 1994; Johnson, Wadsworth, Wellings, and Field 1994.
24. Hamer and Copeland 1998.
25. Ehrlich 2002.
26. Bawer 1994.
27. Hall and Hall 2007; Jenny, Roesler, and Poyer 1994; Murray, J. B. 2000.
28. Clark 2006.
29. Gallup 1995.
30. Heller 2003.
31. Garber 2003.
32. Szymanski 2004.
33. Whitehead 2008.
34. Frost and Meyer 2009.
35. Fortunata and Kohn 2003; McClennen 2005; Ohms 2008.
36. Fortunata and Kohn 2003; Frost and Meyer 2009; McClennen 2005; Ohms 2008.
37. Remafedi, French, Story, Resnick, and Blum 1998; Russell and Joyner 2001; Rutter and Soucar 2002.

38. Plöderl and Fartacek 2009; Ryan, Huebner, Diaz, and Sanchez 2009; Skidmore, Linsenmeier, and Bailey 2006.

39. Ryan, Huebner, Diaz, and Sanchez 2009.

40. Egan, Edelman, and Sherrill 2008.

41. Laumann et al. 1994.

42. Edgar, Edelman, and Sherrill 2008.

43. Acs and Neslon 2003.

44. Cameron 2006; Latham 2005.

45. Stacey and Biblarz 2001.

46. Ibid.

47. Robitaille and Saint-Jacques 2009.

48. Herek n.d.

49. Cameron 2006.

8

Is It a Secret Agenda
or a Civil Rights Movement?

A few years ago, I happened to be in Atlanta the weekend of the city's annual Gay Pride celebration. As I am apt do when visiting the city, I went to the Flying Biscuit diner in Midtown for breakfast. Located on Piedmont and 10th, with the OutWrite Bookstore and Coffeehouse across the corner, the diner sits close to ground zero for Atlanta's gay culture.

Waiting outside for a table to open up inside the diner, a friend and I were surrounded by demonstrators protesting Gay Pride as well as lesbian and gay passersby who were engaging in their own slogan-shouting, yelling taunts at the 15 or so men carrying their antigay posters. At least a few of the demonstrators seemed to belong to a group that had tried to get the local city council to revoke the permit for the Gay Pride Parade that would take place the next day.

In watching the actions and interactions among the two groups, all I could think was, here was our constitution at work—Americans exercising their constitutional rights to free speech by yelling their favorite slogans and retorts at each other, each convinced he or she had a corner market, literally and figuratively, on Truth. Yet, somehow I doubt that anything was added to the ongoing national debate on that particular Saturday. There certainly was no dialogue going on in this exchange of rants and jibes, and nothing that I heard that morning from either side was particularly new or insightful. Instead, I noted that many of the participants exhibited what appeared to be a surface arrogance and hostility likely born of internal fear and self-doubt—the kinds of fear and doubt that might drive you to yell louder when arguing with friend or foe.

Standing there, I also noticed that almost to the person, gay men and lesbians who were in their thirties or older passed by the demonstration with little to no reaction: been there, done that, moving on. It was the late-teen and early-twenties portion of the homosexual contingency that felt impassioned to counter the demonstrators' attacks and prove that they were equipped with the verbal grenades needed to defend their territory: "It's in my genes, you . . ." "If you really understood the Bible . . ." The antigay protestors, on the other hand, were somewhat older than the young gay warriors. Ranging in age from mid-twenties through their forties, these demonstrators seemed just as needy in trying to prove their point—they had found God, and He was personally standing with them as they battled to hold back the demise of civilization.

The message that these protestors were struggling to get across to an audience that refused to listen was essentially the same as what James Dobson, Laura Schlesinger, Pope Benedict, and their fellow travelers have expressed over and over again, often using the label "the homosexual agenda" as the code to describe the evil intent of the gay community:[1] Lesbians and gay men are plotting to radically change the world as we know it. And as part of their secret agenda, these homosexual women and men are seeking to secure special rights for themselves, using propaganda and deceit to recruit others into supporting their cause. If homosexuals, bisexuals, and transgender individuals succeed in fulfilling this agenda, the result of their trickery and debauchery will be the eventual destruction of our society. Make no mistake, the enemy is not an oppressed and underprivileged minority. The enemy is a real force to be reckoned with, and our very way of life is in imminent danger.

The shouts that emanated from the lesbian and gay chorus were, as could be predicted, quite different, echoing the message of organizations such as the Human Rights Commission and Lambda Legal Defense Fund: "We have no secret agenda. All we ask for is to be treated as any other free citizen and to be protected from efforts to deny us our civil and human rights and from those that would eliminate us from the face of the earth." But there on the street, the passion was so much more visible and thus the message so much less cogent. Almost certainly, the only change that took place in Atlanta that June morning was a further hardening of defenses against the evil of the other. Although the histrionics from both sides may have served to reaffirm the opinions within their respective groups, it is unlikely that either side was ready or willing to hear the other. It seemed that these individuals weren't even listening to members of their own group. Instead, the men and women on Piedmont and 10th were engaging in side-by-side monologues, rehearsing their own political gospels, unwilling to learn from each other, but more than willing to outshout the opponent.

WHAT'S IN A NAME?

So what name do we put on efforts to change lesbian, gay men, and bisexuals' legal and social status? Is it a secret homosexual agenda, or is it a fight for civil rights? And why does it even matter which label we use? In choosing our words, we know that contrary to the line Shakespeare gave Juliet, a rose does not necessarily smell as sweet by any other name. And it definitely makes a difference if you are a Capulet or a Montague as to whether you see the flower's beauty or feel its thorns.

In this case the words we choose have come to represent more than a simple stylistic difference; they telegraph our perspectives on the position LGBT individuals hold within the culture. Are we to consider homosexuals or bisexuals as troubled citizens, many of whom are trying to gain unwarranted and potentially dangerous power, or are we to think of them as oppressed individuals who are seeking to become fully functioning and fully integrated members of society? For the antigay conservative leaders among us, the answer to the first question would be a resounding "It's an agenda." From the perspective of the gay and lesbian rights proponents in our culture, there is no agenda, at least as implied by conservative voices, but rather an effort to gain equal protection under the law. Even this disagreement on the terms we use seems fierce at times because the underlying fight has become characterized as a battle of survival—the destruction of society versus the freedom of the oppressed.

With this level of conflict, it is not surprising that each side accuses the other of using unfair tactics in this cultural struggle. Of course, much like the case of the morning melodrama on Piedmont and 10th, both groups seem to be taking moves from the same playbook: characterizing its members as the victims, claiming their liberties have been denied, demonizing the other by linking them to the devils of the past, alleging that their opponents are using political and personal pressure as a substitute for reason and science, and employing propaganda machines to rally the troops.

Men and women who oppose corporate nondiscrimination policies are filing lawsuits, claiming that these policies are limiting their rights to free speech and to dissent against gay and lesbian rights. These policies are imposing a political correctness in the workplace that inhibits the expression of thought. At the same time, homosexuals are taking their turn in court, asserting that human rights protections found in various state constitutions have been violated in child custody cases and by laws that prohibit same-sex marriage. Each side is claiming to be denied their constitutionally guaranteed protections.

In 1992, Ty and Jeannette Beeson, Springs of Life Ministries, produced the first of a series of videos depicting what they titled the Gay Agenda. In this video, leaders from the Christian right explain how gay and lesbians are organizing to normalize homosexuality while using calculated methods to recruit more people into accepting a gay lifestyle. Montages of gay pride demonstrations and parades serve as a backdrop to the testimonials. Most of the scenes include provocatively and outlandishly dressed men and women engaged in activities that call their sense of decorum into question, providing evidence for the judgments made by the self-proclaimed experts (Herman 1997).

Since these videos first appeared, the term *gay [homosexual] agenda* has become code, signaling a view of the gay and lesbian movement as an attempt to usurp the rights of others and impose the collective will of homosexuals on society in general. Examples of this usage range far and wide, including Justice Scalia's dissenting opinion in *Lawrence v. Texas*, the court decision that struck down Texas's homosexual conduct law.

In responding to the use of the term *homosexual agenda*, the Gay and Lesbian Alliance Against Defamation (GLAAD) media reference guide suggests that at least in this context, the term *agenda* has been intentionally distorted, taking on an offensive tone. GLAAD proposes that a better way to understand and characterize what is happening in America is to think of it as an ongoing struggle to secure civil rights, not special rights.

In response to protestations from Gay and Lesbian rights groups, members of the Christian Right correctly point to the fact that the term agenda has been used by different gay and lesbian groups and writers, especially in the 1980s and early 1990s, to describe both the objectives of the gay and lesbian rights movement and the strategies that could be used to achieve these objectives. Two of the most commonly referenced uses of the term come from a 1988 meeting of 175 gay and lesbian activists that was held in Warrenton, Virginia and from a book entitled *After the Ball* (Kirk and Madsen 1989). In *After the Ball*, authors Marshall Kirk and Hunter Madsen detailed a plan to move the gay agenda forward. At the meeting in Warrenton, the participants developed a list of goals, many of which are still central to the gay and lesbian civil rights movement. Some of the goals that came out of this meeting were, however, quite controversial within the gay community at the time and remain so today. These particular goals have been denounced by the majority of gays and lesbians: approval of polygamy and of sex between adults and teenagers.

Not surprisingly, members of the Christian Right use these particular goals as exemplars of why the gay and lesbian rights movement is to be feared. Of course, these members of the Christian Right forget or deny that maintaining racial segregation was a central goal of many churches that are a part of the larger Christian Right movement and that even today, equal rights for women is seen as suspect in several of these churches.

In their political discourse, gay and lesbian rights activists are quick to associate antigay rights leaders with Nazi Germany, where homosexual men were sent to the concentration camps. In turn, conservative leaders equate the tactics of the LGB rights activists with the propaganda and reprogramming of Mao Dzedong. Conservative writers assert that the American Psychiatric Association bent to political pressure instead of following the science when it removed homosexuality from its list of psychiatric disorders. Gay rights scholars tell us that there is no creditable science to support conversion therapies and that hard science does, in fact, support homosexuality as one normal variant of human sexuality. But conservatives are preventing schools and courts from teaching and acting on this science.

The term *sodomy* is typically used when talking about sexual behaviors among homosexuals and in describing anal and oral heterosexual behaviors. Laws that prohibit these behaviors are referred to as the sodomy laws. In this text we use somewhat more cumbersome terms. Laws that ban same-gender sex are called homosexual conduct laws—a term taken from the Texas law struck down by the Supreme Court. Laws that ban anal or oral sex for hetero- and homosexuals are called consenting-adult sexual conduct laws.

The reason for this substitution is that use of the terms *sodomy* and *sodomite* reinforces a cultural assumption that the sin that occurred in the biblical account of Sodom and Gomorrah was sex among men. For more than a millennium, including during the life of Jesus, the sins of Sodom were thought to be gluttony and a lack of caring for strangers. The connection between the sins of Sodom and same-gender behaviors did not occur until 93 C.E., first seen in the writings of a Jewish scholar named Flavius Josephus (1988).

In an attempt to avoid perpetuating what may be an inappropriate and historically inaccurate linkage, I avoid using the words *sodomy* or *sodomite*, despite the fact that it has become the commonly used vernacular. I have no doubt that some readers are likely to pause and utter, "political correctness gone wild."

With all of these charges and countercharges, any one of us could easily find a would-be-expert to confirm our own personal beliefs, no matter what they are. At the same time, unless we live in a highly insulated community, we are also likely to be accosted by opposing voices telling us how misguided we are. So how do we as individuals sort through the arguments and counterarguments to find our own answer to the question: is it a secret agenda aimed at imposing socially destructive rights, or are we looking at a legitimate fight for equal and what should be inherently basic rights? One way is to focus on actual and supposed elements of this agenda, trying to hear both sides on a specific argument and asking basic questions. Following this pattern, let's look at four elements that are central to the fight for equal rights as defined by mainstream LGBT organizations. These four elements include efforts to (a) repeal laws prohibiting same-gender sex, (b) establish laws that prohibit making employment decisions (hiring, firing, promoting an individual) based on sexual orientation, (c) provide domestic partner benefits for same-sex couples, and (d) recognize same-sex marriages. We'll also examine a fifth element that is often mentioned as part of the gay agenda by opponents of gay rights, but one that has been rejected by major LGBT organizations: eliminating laws that prohibit sex between adults and adolescents. A sixth element is discussed in the following chapter: open discussion of gay and lesbian issues in public and postsecondary school curricula. Given that repealing laws that prohibit same-gender sexual activity has already been addressed by the Supreme Court in its *Lawrence v. Texas* decision, this serves as a good place to begin our examination.

THE CAMEL'S NOSE IS UNDER THE TENT

For close to two centuries, up until 1960, every state in the union had a law on its books prohibiting oral and/or anal sexual acts, as did most nations.[2] These sexual conduct ordinances included proscriptions for both opposite-sex and same-sex couples. Rarely, if ever, used in prosecuting consenting heterosexuals, these statutes were pulled from the books on some occasions to make an example of homosexuals. More frequently, they served as a way to drive homosexual behavior into the shadows of society and as the basis for denying LGB men and women other rights and privileges (e.g., employment in certain professions such as teaching, the right to hold common-interest meetings in public forums such as schools and public libraries, the right to dance openly together in gay bars, and equal treatment in the courts when physically attacked for flaunting their sexual deviance). After all, if these individuals were breaking the law in their bedrooms, why would they expect to be treated as fully functioning members of society? Wasn't it enough that they didn't have stormtroopers in their homes? With few gay or bisexual men and no women in court on sexual conduct charges, the real effect of these prohibitions was that LGB citizens understood their place on the margins of society and knew that they were expected to remain silent and in their closets.

Although the majority of nations had laws prohibiting oral and anal sex until the 1960s, this was not true in all instances. France and Belgium repealed their noncommercial, consenting-adult sexual conduct laws in 1790. In the 1800s Brazil, Spain, and Japan also legalized same-gender sex. Japan's prohibition on same-gender sex actually lasted only from 1872 until 1880. Denmark, Sweden, Iceland, and Portugal struck down their laws in the early 20th century (National Gay and Lesbian Task Force n.d).

Among a number of indigenous tribes in Australia and other parts of the globe, there were no prohibitions of these sexual acts. To the contrary, same-gender sex was accepted as a part of the culture (Ford and Beach, 1951).

In 1962 the pendulum began to swing. That year, the State of Illinois repealed its noncommercial, sexual conduct laws for both homosexual and heterosexual couples. These laws had prohibited oral and anal sex between consenting adults. This same year, the nation of Hungary took similar action. Then one by one, the majority of states and most Western nations that still had prohibitions followed suit, eliminating noncommercial sexual conduct laws. By the year 2000, 36 states had removed these laws from their penal codes.

Running contrary to the prevailing trend, Texas took a different course of action. In 1973, the Texas legislature eliminated its law prohibiting anal and oral sex for any couple and replaced it with a homosexual conduct law, prohibiting only same-gender sex. This change in statutes set the stage for a U.S. Supreme Court decision overturning this Texas law and the high Court's own 1986 ruling upholding Georgia's right to forbid anal and/or oral sex between any two people.

On the day the Court handed down its decision, I was in Cleveland visiting my mother. Driving to the nursing home to see her, I was listening to WKSU, a National Public Radio affiliate. As the morning anchor announced the six-to-three decision, tears began streaming down my face. Having lived in Ohio, another state that banned same-sex relationships until I was 29, and then having moved to Florida, for the first time in my life my physical expression of love for my partner was legal. I pulled off the road and cried; no holiday or birthday celebration had or will ever mean as much to me as that moment. I grabbed my cell and called my partner at our home in Florida, a state in which our affection had been illegal until that very day. Another NPR junkie, he answered the call with tears in his voice. As we talked, I fully recognized that there were others, including a few friends and cousins, who were feeling quite a different set of emotions. For them a blazing and potentially fatal stake had been driven into the heart of our society; we were on the road to destruction.

In their 2003 *Lawrence v. Texas* ruling, the Supreme Court said that because the Texas law failed to give due process to homosexuals, it was unconstitutional. The Court went further and set aside all remaining state laws prohibiting oral and anal sexual acts for both homosexuals and heterosexuals, reversing its *Bowers v. Hardwick* ruling. With the Court's *Lawrence v. Texas* decision, America joined most Western countries in declaring the right to engage in same-gender sex, and by extension same-gender love, as a freedom guaranteed to its citizens: "Liberty presumes an autonomy of self that includes freedom of thought, belief, expression, and certain intimate conduct."[3]

With this landmark ruling, American LGB activists celebrated, whereas antigay forces saw it as a major blow to their efforts to keep homosexuality in check. As they had predicted, the camel's nose was more than under the tent. From inside that tent, you could see her entire head, and there was no doubt about it, the camel wanted to come in and join the rest of the crowd.

The impact of this decision had the potential of changing the culture, affecting both the pro– and anti–gay rights contingents. On the day it was announced, gay rights advocates believed that *Lawrence v. Texas* would be the equivalent of *Brown v. Board of Education of Topeka*. From the perspective of conservatives opposed to the acceptance of homosexuality, this decision was an absolutely frightening case of judicial activism that would weaken and, if left unchecked, destroy this country's moral code. The Court had succumbed to the gay agenda, and this meant a call to arms.

In writing for the Court, Justice Kennedy[4] questioned the state's interest in suppressing homosexual behavior and in maintaining a morality code that deprived LGB citizens of the equal protection and due process guaranteed under Section 1 of the Fourteenth Amendment:

All persons born or naturalized in the United States, and subject to the jurisdiction thereof, are citizens of the United States and of the State wherein they reside. No State shall make or enforce any law which shall abridge the privileges or immunities of citizens of the United States; nor shall any State deprive any person of life, liberty, or property, without due process of law; nor deny to any person within its jurisdiction the equal protection of the laws.

The Court's ruling asserted that by making sexual behavior between consenting same-sex partners illegal, the states were regulating the most intimate of human behaviors, invading the privacy of the bedroom, and attempting to control personal relationships. And in doing this, the states and past affirming courts were relying on an empty plea of state interest and what many scholars would say were overly sweeping and flawed historic analyses as the bases for such past decisions.

In offering a minority dissent, Justice Scalia[5] echoed the feelings of many of his fellow conservatives—the Court had gone too far and was not interpreting the Constitution but was rewriting it to fit the will of social activists:

Today's opinion is the product of a Court, which is the product of a law-profession culture, that has largely signed on to the so-called homosexual agenda, by which I mean the agenda promoted by some homosexual activists directed at eliminating the moral opprobrium that has tradition-ally attached to homosexual conduct.

In his dissent, Scalia did not question whether homosexual intimacy was a personal liberty; in fact he stated that it was. But he went on to say that it was not a fundamental right, and therefore, legislatures could regulate this liberty if they deemed it in the best interest of the state, and courts should not presume to pass judgment on these claims of state interest.

In comparing and contrasting these two perspectives, both sides of the Court recognized sexual behaviors between consenting adults as a liberty. But they differed on whether there was a valid state interest in limiting this liberty among homosexuals. The arguments in *Lawrence v. Texas* rested on whether a state had significant interest in prohibiting intimacy among same-sex couples and whether this interest was sufficient to curtail the lib-erty sought by homosexuals and bisexuals constrained by these legislative actions. Scalia argued that tradition and past precedent indicated that the state does have sufficient interest. In contrast, Kennedy questioned Scalia and the earlier *Bowers v. Hardwick* Court's selective use and interpretation of history in determining precedent. In doing so, he provided examples of an overreaching use of past laws written to protect minors as an assumed precedent for regulating same-sex behavior among adults and examples of evolving societal views on homosexuality: that is, the model penal code developed by the American Law Institute and the British Wolfenden Re-port. Kennedy also cautioned that laws prohibiting same-gender behaviors were more often used to censure relationships and nonsexual behaviors among homosexuals than to regulate their sexual activity. In this ruling, Kennedy and his fellow jurists found insufficient state interest to meet the standards set forth in the Fourteenth Amendment.

Both Kennedy and Scalia built their decisions, in large part, on the ques-tion of state interest: Is there sufficient cause to deprive or abridge homo-sexuals of a liberty exercised by other citizens? For Scalia, the Court had no cause to disregard past precedent, which, at least for him, documented this state interest. For Kennedy, past precedent was flawed, and based on current judicial review, these laws had no legitimate purpose. Instead the state interest appeared to be the imposition of a majority morality on a minority group. (See further discussion of state interest in a later section in this chapter.)

WORKING TOWARD FREEDOM

Even today, several years after the *Lawrence v. Texas* decision, many of us who are homosexual and bisexual go to work unsure whether our jobs would be there if our employers found out about our sexual orientation. LGB students in colleges of education are often advised to hide the fact that they are homosexual when applying for teaching jobs in more conservative school districts. And hardworking men and women fear that the next promotion is in part dependent on their staying in the closet. In 30 of the states, these fears are reinforced by the fact that there is no nondiscrimination law protecting bisexual or homosexual employees in private industry, and in 20 states there are no protections in private or state-funded public sector employment.

Employment prohibitions based on sexual orientation have followed a pattern not too dissimilar from the history of restrictions on sexual behavior, with the major exception being that as of today, there are still no federal laws or court rulings that establish a national standard of protection. In the 1940s, 1950s, and 1960s, we find laws and regulations that placed specific prohibitions on the employment of homosexuals and bisexuals: that is, rules that barred homosexuals and bisexuals from working in certain professions and certain areas of government, including, of course, the armed services.[6] And the absence of nondiscrimination laws ensuring equal employment rights meant that individual employers were free to fire or to refuse to hire employees based solely on perceived or actual sexual orientation.

> The Eisenhower order, a response to Senator Joseph McCarthy's now-infamous Senate hearings on communism, placed significant limitations on gays, lesbians, and bisexuals seeking federal employment.
>
> During the McCarthy hearings, homosexuality and communism were erroneously linked: The evil within people (communists) would show up in many facets of their lives (sexual perversions). Of course, communist cultures proved to be even more hostile toward homosexuality than U.S. culture.

Tracking changes in public attitudes, we find that some of these past prohibitions and practices have been eliminated, whereas others have been modified over the last few decades. In the 1970s and 1980s, law and medicine removed prohibitions against licensing gay and lesbian professionals. In the 1990s President Clinton signed an executive order prohibiting discrimination based on sexual orientation in civil employment in the executive branch of the federal government, overturning an order approved by President Eisenhower in 1953.[7] Clinton also used an executive order to change military practices, allowing homosexuals and bisexuals to join the military, with the often-contested proviso that these military personnel couldn't tell anyone about their sexual orientation.

More recently, a growing number of states and local governments have taken even further steps, passing their own statutes and ordinances making discrimination in employment based on sexual orientation illegal. At the same time, the federal government has failed to pass ENDA (the Employment Non-Discrimination Act), a national law that would bar discrimination in public and private employment based on sexual orientation.[8] Taken together, these different actions have left us with a changing and, at times, confusing patchwork of employment laws and practices as related to sexual orientation.

First introduced in Congress in 1994, the ENDA (the Employment Non-Discrimination Act) would set national standards for nondiscrimination in employment based on sexual orientation. Although ENDA doesn't call for affirmative action, it does prohibit discrimination in hiring, firing, promotions, and compensation. The proposed law exempts religious organizations, companies with 15 or fewer employees, and the armed services from its provisions. The law has so far failed to win congressional approval (Human Rights Campaign 2009b).

Twenty states prohibit discrimination in governmental and nongovernmental employment based on sexual orientation.[9] This means that in 30 states, a nongovernment employer can refuse to hire you based on an assumption about or direct knowledge of your sexual orientation. These same employers can also fire or pass you over for promotion because of your sexual orientation. In 10 of these 30 states, although private employers can use your sexual orientation in making employment decisions, if you work for state government, you are protected against employment discrimination. To add to the confusion, in several of the states in which employment decisions can be made based on sexual orientation, local city or county ordinances prohibit employment discrimination based on sexual orientation. For example, although Texas has no employment protections based on sexual orientation, Dallas, the state's largest city, and Austin, the state capital and one of the more progressive cities in the state, both have ordinances prohibiting discrimination in private- and public-sector hiring.

While homosexuals and bisexuals have legal protections against employment discrimination in twenty states, in only ten of these states do these protections extend to individuals based on gender identity (Human Rights Campaign 2009c).

Within the gay, lesbian, and bisexual communities, there is an ongoing discussion as to how closely the rights of persons with different gender identities should be tied to homosexual and bisexual rights. Leading human rights organizations are committed to working for gender-identity rights at the same time and with the same vigor as they campaign for lesbian, gay, and bisexual employment rights. There are, however, a number of instances where LGB individuals have argued that we shouldn't hold up securing rights for the homosexual and bisexual communities until society is ready to extend rights to transgendered and other persons with differing gender identities.

This difference of opinion represents an ongoing struggle within the gay, lesbian, bisexual, and transgender communities.

In addition to the various state, local, and federal laws and regulations, we also find different corporate policies, with growing numbers of corporations creating their own, often more progressive employment practices related to sexual orientation. Close to 90 percent of the corporations included in the Fortune 500 list have nondiscrimination policies that address sexual orientation. Only 30 percent, however, include gender identity in these policy statements.[10]

The public discourse over employment law is far less audible than the often-shrill public debates over domestic partner benefits and same-sex marriage. But the struggle for employment nondiscrimination is a foundation of the ongoing conversation on sexual orientation. For many of us, the fact that an employer could fire or refuse to hire an LGBT individual seems antithetical to our understanding of the inalienable rights to life, liberty, and the pursuit of happiness. For others, the fight for nondiscrimination employment laws is seen as nothing less than seeking special rights for gay, lesbian, bisexual, and transgender individuals.

In these conversations, those among us who talk about special rights imply that if a federal nondiscrimination law passes, it would mean affirmative action in hiring gays, lesbians, or bisexuals or even quotas for the number of homosexuals that must be employed within a company. In reviewing current state or proposed federal law, we find that none of these statutes carry any such provision. These laws are closer to the laws that reference non-discrimination based on religious affiliation. Corporations aren't expected to balance their workforce based on religious preference, but they are prohibited from making judgments about an applicant or employee based on his or her religious beliefs. Similarly, an employer wouldn't be expected or encouraged to seek us out for hire because we were a gay male, a lesbian, or a bisexual person. But under these laws, the employer couldn't deny us a position based on our sexual orientation, with certain exceptions. One such exception is made for employment in religious hierarchies. Our churches, synagogues, or mosques could reject ordaining gays, lesbians, or bisexuals or elevating homosexual or bisexual clergy to leadership roles solely on the basis of the individual's sexual orientation.

These nondiscrimination laws also don't dictate thought. Those who are conservative in our faith could still preach that homosexuality is wrong, just as we can preach that other faiths are wrong. But in a nonreligious work setting, we couldn't refuse to work alongside a homosexual or bisexual, just as we can't refuse to work alongside a coworker of a different faith.

There is no doubt that passing such state or federal laws does "normalize" gays, lesbians, and bisexuals to some degree, but it doesn't mean discriminating against people who believe differently. Rather, it means accepting that we have differences of opinions. It does, however, mean that we move away from treating bisexuals, lesbians, and gay men as criminals and start treating them as the neighbor next door, albeit possibly a neighbor who holds different views than we might.

In a 17-nation survey, Stack and Eshleman (1998) found that married couples reported greater levels of happiness than single people. People who lived together without the benefit of marriage were happier than singles but fell below the levels reported by married couples.

Studying health levels and health-related behaviors of married men versus single men, Mullen (1996) documented that married men showed increased levels of social integration and, in turn, emotional stability in comparison with their single counterparts. And this social integration was associated with improved physical and psychological health. Generally, married men also reported engaging in fewer health-negative behaviors.

Although the benefits of marriage are well researched, these benefits disappear when the marriage deteriorates into a low-quality or unhappy union. In these cases divorced individuals fare better than their married peers (Hawkins and Booth 2005).

In arguing against these laws, many of us say we don't want to discriminate against lesbians, bisexuals, and gay men, but we don't want to be forced into hiring them. LGB people should just be treated like anyone else. Unfortunately, in places where such laws don't exist, it is perfectly legal to refuse to hire someone because of her or his sexual orientation. But in places where laws are on the books, there is no obligation to hire someone because she or he is homosexual or bisexual.

SUPPORTING COMMITTED RELATIONSHIPS

Research suggests that individuals in committed relationships engage in sex with fewer people,[11] and they are likely to live happier, longer, and healthier lives, with greater financial security.[12] Understanding this, it is easy to see why our society would have an interest in supporting committed relationships. In the same vein, if measures of happiness and health increase when the committed relationship is framed in marriage, and if children thrive better in homes with two loving parents, the state's interest in championing marriage becomes even more compelling. With these and other benefits emanating from marriage, the U.S. government has passed or put in place 1,138 different legislative and regulatory provisions that discuss interests related to married couples.[13] Some of these regulations and laws provide support for the emotional bonds of married couples, their parenting rights, and their property rights and financial security.[14] Investing in marriage is good public policy and good politics.

Views on same-sex unions including marriage are changing across the country. While in 2004 the majority of Americans favored a federal constitutional amendment banning same-sex marriage, in 2008, 56 percent of the U.S. population opposed such an amendment. And by a narrow margin, 49 percent to 45 percent of Americans oppose an amendment banning same-sex marriages in their own state constitutions (Quinnipiac 2008). As is true for all Americans, there are changes and differences in opinions on same-sex marriage among gay and lesbian Americans. When gay men and lesbians were asked if they view same-sex marriage rights as an extremely important element of the struggle for civil rights, 52 percent of all respondent said yes. When broken down by age, 75 percent of those between the ages of 18 to 25 said yes, whereas slightly under 50 percent of respondents 65 years or older said yes. Older gays and lesbians were more likely to see hate crimes and workplace discrimination as being more important (Egan, Edelman, and Sherrill 2008).Considering all of the advantages inherent in marriage, including the economic, governmental, and social systems we have organized to support these unions, it should be no surprise that same-sex couples have made domestic partner benefits and same-sex marriage central elements in their fight for equal rights. With marriage as the ultimate goal, these same-sex couples see domestic partner benefits as a stop-gap in securing workplace dividends denied them because they are forbidden to marry. Domestic partner benefits also signal recognition of the fact that the LGB employee's work is of equal value to the work of their heterosexual counterparts. Yet even with these benefits, same-sex couples lack access to the numerous state and federal support systems given to heterosexual married couples.

In the campaign to secure these various advantages, LGB rights activists have made their greatest progress in building the case for domestic partner benefits. Efforts to change marriage laws have met with a great deal more resistance.

Domestic Partner Benefits

The arguments offered in support of domestic partner benefits can be illustrated by a conversation that presents an amalgam of facts drawn from the lives of two different sets of friends of mine who left Florida for positions at California and New York universities that offered domestic partner benefits:

> Hal, I just don't understand why you would leave this university for the offer you're getting in California. There isn't that much difference in the pay, and the difference in the cost of housing should make you stop and think.

> Trust me, John, I have looked at the numbers, and I will be better off at UCLA. You know, my student ratings are the highest in the department, and I have brought in more research dollars in the past three years than anyone else, except for Joe, of course. If this university really appreciated me, I think I would be getting the same or better compensation package than Jennifer. No doubt, she's a great faculty member, but I am bringing more to the university at this point.

> But Hal, your salary is $6,000 higher than Jen's, and I have told you I can bump it up a little; this doesn't make sense.

> Sure, my salary is higher, but Jennifer is able to put her husband and his children and their new baby on her health insurance. She also got two months' paid maternity leave. I can't put Steven on my insur-

ance, and that means he can't stay home when he adopts his sister's son. And with all the medical needs that Brandon has, someone needs to be home with him for the first couple of years. Now, are you going to increase my salary enough to pay for the cost of private health insurance? And am I going to get a leave to stay home when we bring Brandon home?

You know I can't raise your salary that high. That would take you above Joe.

My salary might be higher, but it wouldn't take my total package above his. I would still be making less in total. Do the math—in California I earn an additional $10,000, and I get health insurance for the whole family. Steven can stay at home for two years while we sort everything out with Brandon. And if he can fit it in, Steven will start taking classes for his graduate degree in counseling, paid for by UCLA. So if you were me, would you stay here, or would you go someplace that treats you the same as everyone else?

Each and every day, many of us are choosing which job offer to take based in part on compensation packages that include high-value fringe benefits. And like Hal, many of us who are gay or lesbian are challenging our current employers to show us that our accomplishments are valued as much as those of our heterosexual peers: if I work as hard and produce as well, why shouldn't I be compensated equally?

> The practice of offering domestic partner benefits began in 1982 when the *Village Voice* newspaper and the Canadian Province of Quebec started to offer employment benefits to employees who were involved in committed same-sex relationships. As these benefit packages began to spread from one company to another and from one industry to the next, same-gender couples were becoming more visible and consequently more accepted within the culture (Partners Task Force for Gay and Lesbian Couples 2007).

Interested in attracting new and retaining some of the best and brightest, growing numbers of companies in competitive employment markets are offering domestic partner benefits as a way of staying in the game. As of 2009, 8 of the top 10 and more than 50 percent of all Fortune 500 companies were offering full benefits. Predictably, Wal-Mart, a company with a history for bad health insurance programs for many of its employees, has been one of the two exceptions.[15] In addition to the changing corporate practices, 13 states and more than 140 local governments and more than 300 college and universities, including every top-ranked research university in the nation, offers these benefits.

Early on, the very real and legitimate fear that domestic partner benefits would lead to a greater acceptance of homosexuality led organizations such as the American Family Association (AFA) to denounce corporations that were offering these employment packages. These relatively unsuccessful protests hit a brick wall in 1997. That year, Disney took the plunge, announcing that it too would offer benefits to its employees' same-gender partners. In response to this move, the AFA and related organizations mounted a boycott of Disney's theme parks and movies. The company that had built its reputation on family entertainment should not be serving as a poster company for gay rights. Within three months, it became apparent that the boycott was a complete failure, and the AFA, somewhat bruised, begrudgingly withdrew its ban on Disney theme parks and movies.

In the same year that the Disney boycott failed, LGB rights advocates used a new strategy to broaden the use of domestic partner benefits. That year, San Francisco passed an ordinance forbidding the city from contracting with companies that didn't offer domestic partner benefits. This included national airlines that flew into the city's airport. The city was modifying a technique the federal government had used to support other nondiscrimination initiatives—if you didn't support certain federal practices of nondiscrimination, you couldn't contract with the federal government. Since 1997, New York, Seattle, and Oakland have passed similar mandates. In most instances, these policies went unnoticed because the major companies that were doing business with San Francisco and the other cities were already offering these benefit packages. In those cases where the companies were not already offering these benefits, there were occasional protests, but more often than not, the shift in policy earned strong support from the employees who were impacted. The minute national corporations offered these benefits to their San Francisco or New York–based employees, LGB employees from across the country asked for and, in virtually all cases, received the same benefits.

For those who support the homosexual agenda, until recently all seemed like it was going according to plan. Whether because companies thought it was the right thing to do, they wanted to remain competitive in the marketplace, or they saw it as a requirement of doing business, more and more companies and governmental entities were including same-sex domestic partner benefits in their employment policies. For those who oppose equal rights for gay men, lesbians, and bisexuals, it seemed like this battle was lost—domestic partner benefits were here to stay, and homosexual relationships were gaining broader acceptance. Recently, however, the winds have started to shift slightly, setting the stage for an interesting and emerging set of legal confrontations.

As conservative coalitions crafted anti-marriage amendments for state constitutions, some of these constitutional mandates began to incorporate language that also forbade recognizing any marriage-like status—for example, civil unions. With these amendments in state constitutions, some conservatives and the groups to which they belong have started to bring lawsuits against employers, asking courts to intervene. The remedy that they seek is the discontinuation of the domestic partner benefits because these employment packages confer a marriage-like, or as some would say "marriage-lite," status on lesbian and gay couples.[16] It seems that the judicial activism that conservatives have opposed when it has been used to advance LGB rights now looks like a promising weapon in the conservative arsenal. This leaves all of us with an interesting and ever-changing hodge-podge of laws and court opinions. On one side we have Massachusetts, Connecticut, Iowa, and Vermont issuing marriage licenses for same-sex couples. And then we have the Michigan Supreme Court ruling that domestic partner benefits at state universities violate that state's constitutional ban on same-sex marriage.

Same-Sex Marriages

Homosexual and bisexual men and women who first celebrated domestic partner benefits also recognized their inherent limitations. When Hal left Florida to take a teaching position at UCLA and listed Steven as his domestic partner for purposes of health insurance, UCLA's contributions to Steven's medical insurance became taxable income for Steven. This was not the case for heterosexual married couples, where UCLA's contribution for the faculty member and spouse were both nontaxable. And although Sue left Exxon to work for BP in part so she could take time from work to stay home with her partner Lisa's son when he was sick, in her state Sue couldn't establish legal-parental or guardianship rights for the little boy she was nursing back to health. Some employers and state governments in America might be telling lesbians, gay men, and bisexuals, "We recognize your relationships," but the federal government and many state governments clearly have been saying quite the opposite. Tax and inheritance laws, social security rules and regulations, adoption laws, and a host of other state and federal policies and practices continue to treat homosexual couples as anything but legitimate, loving partners. And the only way to overcome these roadblocks to equality is through legal marriage, recognized by federal and state governments. But until recently, the resistance to this path has seemed insurmountable.

The struggles over same-sex marriage laws represent what may be the ultimate battle for advocates and opponents of the LGB rights movement. For those of us who are advocates, legalizing same-sex marriages means that full equality is sure to follow. For those who are strong opponents, prohibiting same-sex marriage is absolutely necessary if we are to avoid the destruction of our civilization. This fight spreads from our church pulpits and our newspaper editorials to our polling booths, as well as into our courtrooms, legislatures, and executive branches of government.

Reflecting our widely varying views about same-sex marriage, a few state courts have overturned laws prohibiting these unions, citing equal protection guarantees within their state constitutions as the bases for their decisions. In other instances, we have gone to the polls to place prohibitions on same-sex marriage in our state constitutions to block the possibility of similar decisions in our state courts. As a result of these and similarly conflicting actions, we have an extremely fractured legal landscape across America. On one side of this landscape, LGB individuals are marrying, other states are substituting civil unions and domestic partnerships (marriage-lite initiatives) for same-sex marriage, and a few states that have neither marriage nor civil unions are willingly recognizing same-sex marriages performed in other states. In contrast, we see a growing number of states with constitutional amendments prohibiting same-sex marriage and some with state statutes banning both marriage and other types of unions. To add a bit more chaos and confusion, some of the states with laws or constitutional amendments prohibiting same-sex marriage are the same states that recognize marriage-lite initiatives, whereas others extend their constitutional prohibitions against same-sex marriage to prohibit these different forms of domestic partner relationships. In Michigan it is illegal to perform same-sex marriages, and it is illegal for state agencies, including state universities, to offer domestic partner benefits to same-sex partners. In New York it is against the law to perform a same-sex marriage or civil union, but same-sex marriages performed outside the state are fully recognized within the state.

In 1994, the federal government weighed in on the battle on same-sex marriage, passing the Defense of Marriage Act (DOMA). A preemptive law approved when the Hawaiian state court looked as if it would allow same-sex marriages, DOMA barred the federal government from offering any recognition to same-sex marriages, regardless of state laws. DOMA also gave states the right to ignore same-sex marriages performed in other states.

By looking at the numbers of states that fall into each of the above buckets, we can see that early on, most of us voiced overwhelming and strong opposition to the idea of same-sex marriage and other such unions. But this trend appears to be shifting slowly. Public opinion polls indicate that as a nation we are slowly building support for same-sex marriage, and we show even stronger support for civil unions. As support for same-sex marriage or marriage-lite initiatives grows, opposition numbers are declining.[17] But the fight is far from over, the topic remains a hot button in our public and private discourse, and neither advocates nor opponents are in a position to declare victory.

Adelphopoiia, or the religious rite of brotherhood, was a special ceremony performed in both the Roman Catholic and Eastern Orthodox churches in the medieval times. This religious service was used to unite two unrelated same-sex persons, most often men, in a union of brotherhood. In his text *Same-Sex Unions in Pre-Modern Europe*, John Boswell asserts that these rites were used by some same-sex couples as form of a marriage ceremony. In offering his treatise, Boswell points to the similarities between these and heterosexual marriage ceremonies of the time.

One of the prayers used in these ceremonies reads as follows:

> For in joining together in union of love and life, we pray to the Lord. For these servants of God, _____ and _____, and for their union in Christ, we pray to the Lord. That the Lord our God unite them in perfect love and inseparable life, we pray to the Lord. That they be granted discretion and sincere love, we pray to the Lord. (301)

In support of his conclusion Boswell points to individuals in the early church who lived in committed relationships with each other: the apostles Philip and Bartholomew and early church martyrs Serge and Bacchus.

Boswell's description of how the rites were used has been questioned by most Church historians.

When considering same-sex marriage, many of us begin by asking, why we can't just leave marriage the way it has been since the beginning of time—one man and one woman bound together in love, with the intent of raising a family? Although that idyllic image of marriage may be comforting to many of us, it certainly doesn't present a true picture of marriage throughout history. Marriage is and always has been in flux, with changes, both good and bad, showing up at different times and in different cultures. So when we say "let's go back to the good old days," we need to be clear as to what point in history were those good old days—the Old Testament acceptance of polygamy, the many centuries when women had no rights and were treated as little more than property in the marriage contract, before the late 1960s when interracial marriages were against some state laws, or prior to the first Europeans landing on the shores of America, when same-sex marriages were recognized by Native Americans? Marriage changes in response to the attitude and temperament of the culture. Because of these shifts, is it surprising that we would be weighing the advantages and disadvantages of same-sex marriages at this point in human history.

In thinking about the advantages and disadvantages of same-sex marriage, we raise a number of basic questions about the purpose and meaning of marriage. For many, marriage is an institution meant to foster procreation and protect our children, and therefore by extension, we assume a union between a man and woman. When we offer this definition of marriage, those of us who advocate for same-sex marriage raise two key objections. The first has been mentioned earlier in this chapter: Churches and society have defined the purpose of marriage as much more than a union meant to protect children. Marriage is a contract by which two consenting adults pledge devotion and love and through which society recognizes the legal commitment and union between these two people. It is how we build our families with or without children, including those opposite-gender couples who are too old or have chosen not to have children. With marriage comes legal, emotional, and health advantages that are separate from and that extend beyond those associated with raising children. Wouldn't we be better off as a society to encourage same-sex partners to make the same declaration of mutual support and interdependence? Ought we deny them the benefits and support systems that come with marriage?

The second objection rests on the idea that if marriage is meant to protect children, shouldn't we use it to protect the increasing number of children who are being raised in gay and lesbian households? Each year, more lesbian and gay couples are assuming joint responsibility for co-parenting children. In many of these cases, one or possibly both partners have biological children that are part of the couple's family. These children may be the result of a prior heterosexual marriage or relationship, or they may be from births involving sperm donors or surrogate mothers. In other cases the children become a part of the family as a result of adoption. With the differences in state adoption laws, many of the children being raised by two same-sex parents are legally related to only one of these parents.

According to the 2000 U.S. Census, that year, 46 percent of married heterosexual couples and 43 percent of unmarried heterosexual couples were raising children. That same year, 34 percent of female couples and 22 percent of male couples were raising children. This pattern of increasing numbers of same-sex couples raising children was true across the country. Surprisingly, the highest rates were in the South.

As same-sex couples join together in raising their children, they want to provide their children with the same advantages and protections children raised in loving heterosexual households have. These same-sex couples want their children to be raised in financially secure homes. They want to provide their children with the protection and love of two parents. And they want their children to integrate into society. As with most parents, these couples are willing to do everything it takes to make these goals a reality. But even under the conditions we hope for in all parent–child relationships, with two healthy and committed parents seeing the child into adulthood, there are more obstacles to achieving each of these goals if marriage is not a part of the equation. Without marriage, a host of financial and societal benefits are taken off the table or become more tenuous and difficult to achieve: the option to have one parent stay home during the formative years; access to the best health care plan offered by the parents' different employers; the ability for either parent to represent the child in legal, medical, and educational decisions; the protection of state-governed inheritance rights if the non-biological/non-adoptive parent dies; flow of custody if the biological/adoptive parent dies; child support if one parent leaves; and so on. Without legally binding marriage, each of these and many other benefits are placed at risk. This is why those of us who are gay and lesbian rights advocates wonder why, if society believes marriage is meant to protect children, shouldn't society be concerned with protecting children being raised by same-sex couples?

In his book *Marriage under Fire,* James Dobson gives voice to a strongly held objection to legalizing same-sex marriage. Dobson contends that such unions would weaken or diminish heterosexual marriage. In making this claim, Dobson offers a number of different assertions linking same-sex unions to the end of marriage as we know it, including the threat of increased promiscuity within marriage and the further spread of HIV. He also presents an argument that polygamous forms of marriage would inevitably follow on the heels of same-sex marriage.[18] There are also some gay men and lesbians who oppose same-sex marriage but for the exact opposite reason. For these homosexuals and bisexuals, the fear is that with same-sex marriage, bisexuals, gay men, and lesbians will adopt a heterosexual ethic and pattern their lives after married heterosexuals, losing the liberation they gain from living outside the norm.[19] From these different sources we have two dissenting reasons for why same-sex marriage is bad—one tells us that heterosexual marriages will be ruined by same-sex marriage because they will take on characteristics often associated with gay males, and the other tells us that gay and lesbian lifestyles will be ruined by same-sex marriage because they will be patterned after heterosexual lifestyles.

Most proponents of same-sex marriage believe that legalized marriage is more likely to have the effect predicted by the queer theorists than the one suggested by Dobson. Several moderate Christian and other conservative writers have suggested that if as a society we find promiscuity to be offensive, we should be encouraging gay men, in particular, to engage in same-sex marriage as a way to socially support monogamous relationships. It seems wrongheaded or at least shortsighted to say we condemn the lifestyle you are leading, but we will not give you the right to enter a relationship that we believe would be better. These writers suggest that if marriage provides a framework for a healthier lifestyle, why wouldn't we encourage gay men and lesbians to adopt this family pattern?[20]

One last question about forbidding same-sex marriage rests on religious freedom. If a church feels it is God's will to sanction the marriage of two-same sex partners, how does the state stand in opposition to this union? Are we denying gay men and lesbians the religious freedom given to others in our society, and on what legal basis do we do so? Marriage is not just a governmental institution; it is a sacred institution, presumably guaranteed to all religions.

STATE INTERESTS

In all of our social battles on marriage and sex, those of us who oppose change have suggested that there are tensions between state interest and individual liberties and that state interest should prevail. This was certainly true in all of the Supreme Court battles on sexuality and marriage: for example, *Loving v. Virginia*—the 1967 decision that struck down laws barring interracial marriage; *Griswold v. Connecticut*—the 1965 ruling that removed laws prohibiting the sale of contraceptives to married couples; and *Einstadt v. Baird*—the 1972 decision that declared laws barring the sale of contraceptives to unmarried couples. This claim was even louder in cases involving the civil rights of bisexuals and homosexuals. Those of us who oppose today's gay, lesbian, and bisexual initiatives are vehement in our assertions that extension of personal liberties to same-sex couples threatens the fabric of society, along with the personal and religious liberties of those opposed to these initiatives. The contention is that by giving rights to homosexuals and bisexuals, we will be giving the devil free reign and depriving heterosexuals of their freedoms.

The passion is equal on the other side of the argument. Those of us who support personal liberty posit that the failure to move forward on these initiatives means that homosexuals and bisexuals continue to be denied their "inherent and inalienable rights [of] . . . liberty and the pursuit of happiness." We ask how and why states have the right to dictate whom we can and can't love.

Those who oppose the gay agenda believe that cultural and legal acceptance of homosexuality means increasing numbers of people living a homosexual lifestyle, weakening the general morality, which in turn will lead to the inevitable destruction of our society. As discussed in chapter 6, "The Downfall of Society," opponents of the gay agenda tell tales of past civilizations that accepted and even celebrated same-sex relationships and how these cultures were destroyed as a result of this "immorality," with the Roman Empire and Classic Greece serving as the oft-cited exemplars. In fighting gay rights, opponents continue by contrasting the history of these "fallen" cultures against a chronicle of an America built on a strong moral foundation and Christian principles, an America that is now threatened by its own growing immorality. Advocates for bisexual and homosexual rights offer a much different picture—a history in which culture, science, and political life advanced in an atmosphere of openness where expression of same-gender love was accepted. In projecting into the future, advocates suggest that instead of destruction, we are sowing the seeds of an open and accepting society in which all people can flourish. As documentation of this belief, advocates focus our attention on the historic and contemporary accomplishments of gay, lesbian, and bisexual members of this and other cultures. Predictably, both of these accounts are self-serving, and the key elements included in the accounts are subject to debate.

Throughout history there have been periods spanning several centuries during which same-gender sex has found varying degrees of acceptance in prospering and innovated societies—including China, Japan, Rome, Greece, and America before the European invasion. And as documented by scholars, none of these societies, including Rome and Greece, collapsed under the weight of homosexual behaviors. In stark contrast to historic periods of acceptance, we find that governments that were or are the least tolerant of homosexual behavior are cultures that have fallen far short of idyllic models for emulation: Nazi Germany, the Soviet Union under Stalin, Communist China under Mao Zedong, and present-day Iran. But lest we be lulled into illusions about those societies that were accepting of same-sex relationships, we should remember that they often had their own outcasts and second-class citizens, including heterosexual, bisexual, and homosexual women. And in some of these societies, adult males who assumed a passive role in sex were looked at with a disdain that reflected the cultural view of women.

Although the underpinnings of conservative fears are founded on bad history, the prediction that more people will adopt a homosexual lifestyle when society accepts this lifestyle, at first glance, appear to be true. Indeed, more men and women seem to be freely acknowledging their homosexuality and bisexuality, with increasing numbers living openly in same-sex relationships. It is important to understand, however, that this increased visibility doesn't mean people are converting to homosexuality. But there certainly is little doubt that greater numbers of homosexuals and bisexuals are becoming more self-aware and more open about their sexual orientation. Instead of more people living a homosexual lifestyle, it is likely that the homosexual lifestyle is changing and becoming more visible. When you remove the stigma of being a criminal in the bedroom, and when the media begins to show you in a positive light, you become free to live an open, healthier, and more self-affirming life. When you are threatened, your lifestyle becomes one lived in the shadows and on the margins.

A compelling case disproving the belief that past societies crumbled as a result of homosexual sex is easily built, as is the case dispelling the prediction that there will be more homosexuals if same-gender sex is accepted within society (see chapter 6, "The Downfall of Society"), but what of the prophecy of a general moral decay within the society? Doesn't society have a right to protect itself from immorality?

Level 1—A Sin against Nature

In drawing the link between homosexuality and societal immorality, those who oppose the homosexual agenda often lay out a series of escalating arguments. At the first level, they offer the thesis that same-gender sex is a sin against nature. That is, same-gender sex is an unnatural form of human sexuality that is made even more sinful by the fact that is inherently non-procreative. And after all, procreation is the reason for sex.

Do heterosexuals engage in non-procreative sex? The answer seems to be a resounding yes. In a survey of 18,876 English men and women ranging in age from 16 to 59 years old, 64 percent of married men and 58 percent of married women reported in engaging in oral sex with their spouse at some point during the previous year. Among unmarried couples living together, 88 percent of men and 79 percent of women reported engaging in oral sex with their partners. Rates of masturbation were similar to the rates for oral sex.

In 1976, 10 percent of married women in the United States remained childless at the age of 44; by 2004, this number had climbed to 19 percent (Johnson, Wadsworth, Wellings, and Field 1994).

Alan Medinger and Wynema Barber, leaders in the ex-gay movement, suggest that masturbation focusing on heterosexual fantasies would be acceptable therapeutic behavior for gay men and lesbians involved in reparative therapy as long as the fantasies do not become obsessive (Medinger 2000, p. 217; Erzen 2006).

The growing body of research on the sex lives of rams, bonobos, gulls, whales, and an ever-increasing host of animals, along with research on sexual orientation among humans, punctures some serious, and for some of us fatal, holes in the assumption that same-gender sex is an unnatural expression of human sexuality. Some birds do it, and some bees do it, as do some humans. Animal anthropology documents that same-gender sexuality is a part of the animal kingdom's sexual spectrum (see chapter 3, "The Origins of Sexual Orientation").

As to whether non-procreative sex is immoral, our contemporary society has made clear that this question must be decided by the individual consenting adults without the police officer in the bedroom, unless, of course, the police officer is one of the consenting adults. Most of our current cultural norms support the proposition that in certain relationships consensual sexual activity can serve to enrich our lives in ways separated from procreation. On one end of what constitutes a very wide continuum of beliefs, there are some of us who suggest that the physical pleasure and afterglow associated with sex may be sufficient reason for the act itself. On the other end of this continuum, others among us allow that sex can serve to enhance companionship and communication as well as provide a physical expression of love between two people, but it must occur within the context of heterosexual marriage. Within these varying opinions, we find specific arguments for intentionally separating sexual activity from procreation, including the belief that it's not the right time to have children, a desire to avoid transmission of inherited or transmissible diseases, and a wish to avoid pregnancy in individuals who don't have the capacity or disposition to parent.[21]

Although each of the positions on this continuum provides a very different view as to the purposes of sexual activity, each allows for sexual activity to be separated from procreation. The most conservative of our views on separating sex from procreation are highlighted by our acceptance of sexual activity among postmenopausal and infertile heterosexual married couples[22] and in the Catholic Church's advancement of natural family planning (i.e., the rhythm method) for married couples.

In considering these perspectives, it is apparent that the most conservative of our peers are arguing not about whether there are times that it might be appropriate to have sex without the possibility of procreation, but rather about who has the right to do this (i.e., heterosexual married couples) and what methods we should use in avoiding or preventing pregnancy (e.g., the rhythm method versus other forms of birth control).[23] An additional criterion that the Catholic Church and other conservative groups impose in defining when sexual activity can be disassociated from procreation is the nature of the sexual act itself (vaginal-penile intercourse versus masturbatory, oral, or anal sex).[24]

The increasing numbers of heterosexual married couples in our society who choose to remain childless and the lower birthrates in the United States, Europe, and parts of Asia, as well as the increasing use of birth control among both married and non-married couples,[25] provide compelling evidence of our collective and growing willingness to separate sex from procreation and to reject many of the doctrines of conservative faiths. This collective willingness has been affirmed by the Supreme Court in its Gris-wold decision, which struck down the Connecticut law that banned the use of contraceptives among married couples and the Einstadt decision that extended the right to use birth control to unmarried couples. *Lawrence v. Texas* further extends the rights of individuals, both hetero- and homosexual, to engage in non-procreative sexual acts.

In providing legal access to birth control to married and unmarried couples, and in striking down noncommercial, consenting-adult sexual conduct laws, the Court was not judging the morality of these acts. Instead, the prevailing justices were saying that because these acts affected only the individuals involved, the decision to engage in any of these behaviors was a matter of individual conscience. With each of these decisions, the Court slowly backed out of the bedroom, telling us that government didn't belong in the sex lives of consenting adults.

Level 2—The Sin of Promiscuity

Although the first level of argument on the morality of same-gender sex rests on the belief that these behaviors are a sin against nature, the next level of argument shifts the focus to questions of promiscuity. In these second-level arguments, our attention is drawn to the fact that gay males have more, and at times strikingly more, sexual partners in the course of their lifetimes than do their straight peers.[26] (See chapter 7.) With this as a documented fact, people opposed to increased liberties for gay men and lesbians will often ask, "If homosexuals are going to act like animals, why would we sanction and thereby encourage these behaviors? Why wouldn't we try to limit or control this immorality?"

In considering this question of why society wouldn't try to control the sexual exuberance of homosexuals, it is important to remember that it is male homosexuals who have the bad rap on this; lesbians are much more like their heterosexual sisters than their gay or straight brothers.

When we take a closer look at the greater numbers of sexual partners gay men may have in their lifetime, we find that this is most likely a multifaceted phenomenon, in part related to gender and to the lack of societal support for commitment. The importance of gender in determining the number of sexual partners becomes apparent when we note that both straight and gay males report thinking about sex more frequently than lesbian or straight females. As an assumed consequence of this reported difference in libido, men also tell researchers that they have had more sexual partners than do women, regardless of sexual orientation. This must mean there are a few heterosexual women who are much busier than the majority. When we analyze this idea that men have a more active libido, we find that if Bill and Bruce, the objects of John's desire, are also thinking about sex as much as John is, it is not surprising that John will score more often than his straight brother Harry, who is thinking about Jill and Joan, who have other things on their minds.

A second variable that influences the number of sexual partners is relationship status. Regardless of sexual orientation, males and females who are in committed relationships report having fewer sexual partners than peers who are not in long-term relationships. But gay males are less likely to be in committed relationships than their straight peers. Parenthetically, we should also note that although men in committed relationship have fewer partners, they report engaging in sexual activity more often than their single peers. It's more likely you will have sex when you live with your partner than it is if you have to search out a new partner each time.

Considering these data, is it really that surprising that gay males have more sexual partners (albeit not necessarily more sex) than their straight counterparts? The focus of their attention, other gay males, are also more driven to have sex, and the society in which these men live is far from encouraging or supportive of committed same-sex relationships. What seems ironic is that gay males are criticized for being promiscuous, and then their sexual escapades are used as a reason to deny them legally sanctioned relationships that could well modify the sexual behavior that offends their critics: "because you are promiscuous, you can't be given the right to enter into monogamous marriages."

Level 3—Legalizing Sex with Minors

After pointing to promiscuity among gay males, those who feel that equal rights for LGB individuals is tantamount to legalizing immorality will often draw connections between homosexuality and pedophilia. Coupling homosexuality with pedophilia has become more common with the spate of Catholic priests on trial for child abuse.[27] In raising their arguments on morality and society, the American Family Association and the Family Research Council also point to the efforts of the North American Man/Boy Love Association (NAMBLA) to legalize sex between adults and adolescents. When NAMBLA's posture on sex with minors is pointed out, at least some of us are led to believe that NAMBLA's clearly stated goal is yet one more part of the gay and lesbian rights movement.

In responding to this argument about the immorality of same-gender sex, supporters of equal rights suggest that we need to disentangle pedophilia from homosexuality and separate NAMBLA's calls to lower the age of consent from the mainstream gay agenda. We also need to understand that pedophilic, incestuous, and other sexual attacks on infants are different from sexual relationships between post-pubescent adolescents and adults, although all of these acts raise grave and legitimate concerns in our society.

An interesting and illustrative comparison can be made contrasting our public and private reactions to the child molestation scandals in the Catholic Church and those that occurred among the members of the Fundamentalist Church of Jesus Christ of the Latter Day Saints. In both cases we were outraged by the behaviors of the adult perpetrators and pained by the plight of the victims. But when we tried to unpack what had happened in these different cases, many of us found ourselves offering very different explanations that may be more telling about our own biases than about the terrible realities that caused these horrendous events. Some of us attributed cause to rampant homosexuality in the priesthood of the Catholic Church. But we didn't assume that it was rampant heterosexuality in the case of Warren Jeffs and his followers. For some of us, Jeffs represented all Mormons, not just his sect. For others of us, the scandals in Texas provided an example of the evils of religious fundamentalism in general and were not confined to the Mormon Church. It seems that our attribution of cause is often a reflection of our political philosophies and out personal boogeymen.

For those of us who are bisexuals, lesbians, or gay men, our stomachs turn every bit as much as our heterosexual sisters and brothers when we read news accounts of pedophilia and other forms of child molestation. But when those of us who are homosexual or bisexual read these stories, we may hold our breath a little bit longer, hoping that this won't be a case of same-gender abuse. This additional pause isn't because we feel less outrage over the little girl cruelly attacked by an adult male, but because we know that every time it is an adult male attacking a little boy or, even rarer, an adult female attacking an underage girl, the stereotype is reinforced—homosexuals are pedophiles. The data, of course, show that there are significantly more adult-male attacks on young girls than any of the other possible combinations (see chapter 7).[28] But when the adult male attacks the innocent little girl, the despicable act doesn't lead to or reinforce a stereotype of the heterosexual male as a pedophile. In these cases, as a society, we fully understand that there are very few straight men who commit these crimes and that these attacks have nothing to do with normal adult sexual behavior. Unfortunately, similar truths are often lost when the story is about an adult male sexually molesting a young male child. For some of us these stories reinforce beliefs that gay men are more likely to be pedophiles and that these behaviors are a normal part of gay sex. Both beliefs, of course, are untrue, even if they are constantly raised by opponents to equal rights for lesbians, gay men, and bisexuals.

LOWERING THE AGE OF CONSENSUAL SEX: IS IT PART OF THE HOMOSEXUAL AGENDA?

But what of NAMBLA's call to legalize consensual sex between adults and post-pubescent adolescents? Isn't this part of the gay agenda, and isn't this a threat to our morality? Early on in the gay liberation movement, members of NAMBLA were vocal and, at various times, influential voices in the struggle for equal rights. Founded in 1978, nine years after Stonewall, NAMBLA and its members were on the frontlines of the gay pride parades, often becoming the focal point for stories that appeared on the evening news. They were also present when coalitions of gay, lesbian, and bisexual groups met, and they were advocating vehemently for a change in age of consent laws.[29] As time moved on, however, so did the LGB rights movement. As the movement matured, it loudly and clearly disassociated itself from NAMBLA, eliminating any reference to proposals to change age of consent laws.[30] The majority of the members of the lesbian, gay, and bisexual rights movement refused to continue their association with what was becoming known as a radical fringe element. In this same time frame, NAMBLA itself began to disassemble. Although it had always been a small organization, it became smaller and smaller, disbanding local chapters and becoming little more than a Web site.

Despite the very visible schism between NAMBLA and the mainstream lesbian, gay, bisexual rights movement, NAMBLA's controversial views remain a hot-button issue in the struggle for equal rights. Conservative opponents of lesbian, gay, and bisexual rights continue to raise the question: won't equal rights for gay men provide them with the license to have sex with teenage boys? The answer to this question may best be given in the form of a set of somewhat related questions: Does the guarantee of religious freedom mean that males in fundamentalist sects of Latter Day Saints and other Christian and non-Christian religious groups have the right to have sexual and, at times, incestuous consensual relationships with underage girls? Or does religious freedom allow certain conservative Christians and other religious faiths to engage in beating children in the name of discipline? I presume the answer is no on all counts. Age of consent laws are and will remain separated from decisions about equal employment rights for homosexuals, domestic partner benefits, or any of the other causes included on the gay agenda, just as laws on incest and laws on child abuse remain separated from this country's clear mandates for religious freedom.

In denouncing *Brown v. Topeka,* the Supreme Court decision that outlawed segregation in schools, Jerry Falwell, founder of the Moral Majority and Liberty University, said,

If Chief Justice Warren and his associates had known God's word and had desired to do the Lord's will, I am quite confident that the 1954 decision would never have been made. The facilities should be separate. When God has drawn the line of distinction, we should not attempt to cross that line.

—Curry 2007

The insistence that the mainstream LGB rights agenda must, at least secretly, include lowering the age of consent because members of NAMBLA marched in gay rights parades and exerted influence on the early gay liberation movement is somewhat like saying that today's conservative Christians are, at least secretly, racists because early leaders of conservative Christianity such as Reverend Jerry Falwell claimed the Bible demanded segregation.

If history provides us examples of periods when same-sex behaviors openly blossomed in thriving and growing societies, if biology tells us that same-sex behaviors are part of the sexual repertoire of most, if not all, animal species, and if same-sex behaviors can be one way to express love and commitment between consenting adults, is there really a state interest in eliminating these behaviors? If some of the most repressive cultures in history were the most effective in pushing same-sex behaviors underground, if a lack of public acknowledgment and acceptance means greater promiscuity, and if hiding one's sexual orientation causes major mental health issues to the closeted individual, is the state interest furthered by prohibiting same-sex behaviors?

The Rest of the Agenda

Decriminalizing same-gender sexual activity, enacting employment non-discrimination laws, and offering the protections associated with same-sex marriage are seen as central to most LGB rights organizations' fight for equal rights. But they are not the only initiatives put forward by these organizations. Many who have been struggling for gay, lesbian, and bisexual rights point to a need for changes in adoption and child custody laws—changes that protect the children of homosexual and bisexual parents and honor the sanctity of committed same-sex relationships. Some of these voices also tell us that we need educational standards and practices that address the needs of lesbian, gay, and bisexual students in schools (these issues are addressed in chapter 9). We also have been fighting for laws that ensure the safety of homosexuals and bisexuals—for example, the recently approved federal hate crimes law—and assurances that equal justice is meted out when a crime is committed against a gay or lesbian citizen, the same as when a crime is committed against a heterosexual citizen. And the list goes on, including overturning Don't Ask, Don't Tell.

But not all gays, lesbians, or bisexuals will agree on these issues. When we ask any two people what should be included and what should be the focus of this agenda, we shouldn't be surprised to get two different answers. The same is, of course, true when we talk about a black agenda, a feminist agenda, a fundamentalist Christian agenda, a Republican agenda, or a Democratic agenda. Individuals within the target group will disagree with each other, as will people from outside the group. When speaking about the gay, lesbian, and bisexual agenda, some would exclude a number of the varying rights and protections advocated by mainstream gay and lesbian organizations for differing reasons. As we have discussed before, a few believe that gays and lesbians are wrongly attempting to adopt heterosexual lifestyles while ignoring the need to assert an independent identity. Others assert that lesbians and gays are hurting themselves by demanding too much, too fast. Some of those who feel that the lesbian, bisexual, gay rights movement is pushing too hard may hold a negative view about their own homo- or bisexuality, convinced that they don't deserve the same rights as heterosexuals (internalized homophobia). Still others fear that there will be a backlash if the gay, lesbian, and bisexual communities are too aggressive: "Couldn't we just accept domestic partner benefits or civil unions and forget marriage?" "Is it necessary to include homosexuality in the school curriculum—isn't silence on the topic sufficient?" "If we move too quickly, are we going to alienate straight allies?"

Although the FBI collects data on hate crimes based on sexual orientation, until recently federal law didn't support prosecution of hate crimes based on sexual orientation.

In the brutal murder of James Byrd, an African American Texan who was dragged out of town by a rope tied to a pickup truck, the federal government spent $300,000 to help the small town of Jasper, Texas, prosecute Byrd's murders because the crime was racially motivated.

In the brutal murder of Matthew Shepherd, a gay American who was beaten and left to die hanging on a fence outside of Laramie, Wyoming, the city government had to lay off five law enforcement officers to cover the cost of prosecuting Matthew's killers because hate crime laws did not cover crimes committed because of sexual orientation (Library of Congress n.d.).

In considering the warnings from those of us who fear we are moving too fast and have become too militant, I am reminded of Martin Luther King's letter from the Birmingham jail.[31] In this letter, King was responding to a letter he had received from a group of moderate white clergymen who were questioning his insistence on conducting the march on Birmingham. King asked these clergymen how long African Americans were supposed to wait for justice, stating that he couldn't "wait for a more convenient season."

Challenged about the cost of the actions he was taking, King responded that action didn't create tension but only brought the already-existing tensions to the surface, forcing us to acknowledge and address them.[32] King strongly rejected the idea that passage of time would solve the problems without direct action.

In the same vein, we could ask how much longer we should expect children to go to schools where they are taunted and put down. How much longer can we allow those who victimize gays and lesbians to go into court and offer a defense that they were so enraged by the behavior of the victim that they were unable to control their actions? How many more times can a judge deny a gay or lesbian caretaker the right to adopt a child the caretaker has supported, loved, and protected? How many more Americans can voluntarily go to war and be killed defending freedoms of others when they must remain silent about loving someone of the same sex? How much longer can those in power impose their standards on this minority group?

Straight Talk

Is there a secret homosexual agenda? No, it's far from a secret. But if we want to label it an agenda, we certainly can. And if we want to label it a civil or human rights movement, we can do that too. Whatever we label it, it's important to remember that others have their own agenda or movement, some of which stands in direct opposition to LGB rights.

The homosexual agenda does not and never did include a call for hiring quotas or targets. And although there were people in the history of the LGB rights movement who did call for the lowering of the age of consent, you will find no mainstream or well-respected gay, lesbian, or bisexual organization that would support that as part of this movement. Nor does the LGB rights movement advocate pedophilia or polygamy. If you want to hold on to the memory of those calls to lower the age of consent, please remember to hold on to the calls of the religious right opposing desegregation.

Many of the items on the agenda are basic rights that most of America believes homosexuals and bisexuals either should or already do have: for example, protection from discrimination in the workplace and housing and the right to join the military. Some of the items are still seen as controversial and lack a majority consensus, such as same-sex marriage. The pleas for the LGB community to accept the gains they have already made and allow some time to go by before pushing for other rights resonate with some members of the LGB community, but certainly not the majority—justice delayed is justice denied.

NOTES

1. Dobson 2007; Robertson 2007.
2. National Gay and Lesbian Task Force (n.d.).
3. Kennedy 2003.
4. Ibid.
5. Scalia 2003.
6. Griffin and Ouellett 2003; Hull 2005.
7. U.S. Department of Personnel Management n.d.
8. Human Rights Campaign 2009b.
9. Human Rights Campaign 2009c.
10. Human Rights Campaign 2009a.
11. Laumann, Gagnon, Michael, and Michaels 1994; Johnson, Wadsworth, Wellings, and Field 1994; Schmitt 2006.
12. Hawkins and Booth 2005; Myers and Scanzoni 2005, 11–22; Popenoe 2007.
13. Shah 2004.

14. Wald 2001.

15. Human Rights Campaign 2007.

16. Jaschik 2008.

17. Quinnipiac University Polling Institute 2008; Hecht 2008; Egan, Edelman, and Sherrill 2008.

18. Dobson 2007.

19. Ettlebrick 2004

20. Brooks 2004; Myers and Scanzoni 2005.

21. Cole and Cole 1999; Ailey, Marks, Crisp, and Hahn 2003 Cassidy 2006; Kemkes-Grottenthaler 2003.

22. Salzman and Lawler 2006.

23. Cones 2006.

24. U.S. Census Bureau 2006; Mencimer 2001.

25. Bensyl, Iuliani, Carter, Santelli, and Gilbert 2005; "U.S. Catholics Still Back Birth Control" 2006.

26. Laumann, Gagnon, Michael, and Michaels 1994; Johnson, Wadsworth, Wellings, and Field 1994; Schmitt 2006.

27. Clark 2006.

28. Jenny, Roesler, and Poyer 1994.

29. Kirk and Madsen 1989.

30. Radow 1994.

31. King 1964

32. King 1964, 87.

9

Out of the School Closet

Having spent all but the first five years of my life in school as student, teacher/professor, and administrator, I have had more opportunities than most to observe the role that education plays in our lives. Although the impact of school doesn't outweigh the contributions of our home and neighborhood, there is no doubt that the explicit and hidden school curricula influence who we are and how we view ourselves. Young elementary school students learning math from a teacher who knows her material and engages her students in active, hands-on learning will certainly be better prepared to pursue careers in math and engineering than if they had been taught passively by an inexperienced teacher who is uncomfortable with mathematics. High school students given the opportunity to work with counselors who guide them to college have a much higher probability of admission to a school of their choice. Undergraduate students working on research projects alongside faculty mentors have an increased chance of pursuing graduate studies. The school's explicit curriculum (course content) can shape how we understand the world around and within us. The school environment (hidden curriculum) can build us up or help tear us down. These are not necessarily the most central forces in our development, but they are critical elements in our socialization.

As is true for all students, lesbian, gay, and bisexual students' understanding of self is influenced by what they do or don't learn in the school setting. The school's decision to ignore or include sexual orientation and same-sex behavior, positively or negatively, in the curriculum has a direct impact on how the students see themselves. Likewise, how these students are treated in the school setting by peers and professional staff and the support systems that address or fail to address the students' unique needs will add to or diminish their emotional and intellectual growth. The availability of a gay–straight alliance (a pro-gay student association) tells Tammy and Sam that the school thinks they belong in the society. The extension of anti-bullying and harassment rules to cover LGB students also helps Tammy and Sam understand that they are safe within the school setting. Silence on the part of the school reinforces the need to remain hidden. Negative messages tell Tammy and Sam to fear society or to be ashamed of themselves. The school's choice to ignore, affirm, or denigrate the LGB student is thus more of an ethical than an educational decision—an ethical decision influenced by political, social, and individual standards.

One set of data that has been used to support greater support for bisexual and homosexual students is the studies on suicide/suicide attempt rates among adolescents. Most of these studies indicate that gay, lesbian, and bisexual youth are at greater risk of suicide than are their heterosexual counterparts (Remafedi, French, Story, Resnick, and Blum 1998; Russell and Joyner 2001; Rutter 2002).

For many of us, these suicide rates document the difficulty LGB adolescents face in acknowledging their sexual orientation in a society that says this part of their being should be denied, changed, or hidden. In response to this hypothesized link between the acceptance of sexual orientation and suicide, a number of people have suggested that schools must provide better information and support for these students.

In contrast, there are others among us who say that the increased rates only prove that homosexuality and bisexuality are a disease that weakens the overall character of the individual. The way to solve the problem is to provide programs to rehabilitate these young men and women. Thus, supportive schools won't help solve the problem; they will only make it worse.

Across America we hold polar-opposite views on how the school ought to address these issues of sexual orientation in the formal and hidden curricula. For some of us the educational system should be labeling homosexuality as deviant. And if schools can't do that, they should at least remain silent on the topic, letting church and home provide the message. To do anything else is tantamount to encouraging moral decay. For others of us, silence is equal to washing our hands of responsibility for some of the most vulnerable of our children. Denigrating or ignoring these students is to cast a pall over their educational experience. Instead schools ought to fully educate and support these students, helping them understand the possible origins of their sexual orientation and the fact that lesbians, bisexuals, and gay men have contributed to many of civilization's greatest achievements.

Acknowledging these different views, school administrators walk a tightrope when forced to make decisions about sexual orientation and school operations. One group or another will criticize, with passion, any course of action a school administration follows. Nonetheless, a decision is inevitably made, even if it is for the school to be silent—the choice most commonly made in today's schools.

SCHOOL TOLERANCE AND SAFETY

We can divide administrative decisions on sexual orientation into three categories: tolerance and safety, supportive environment, and the formal curriculum. The most basic and telling of these may be the decisions on tolerance and safety: Do schools commit to protecting the safety of lesbian, gay, and bisexual students, not by inference but by an explicit statement and specific practices?

Although almost all schools have safe-school or anti-bullying policies, these policies are more often than not silent about issues specifically related to gay, lesbian, or bisexual students. Less than 40 percent of these policies include direct reference to protection based on sexual orientation. In contrast, 66 percent of these schools reference racial and religious differences in their policies (Harris Interactive 2008).

When we ask the question, "Does your school have a program to protect gay, lesbian, and bisexual students from harassment and physical harm?" we will hear several different answers, with the majority sounding something like this: "This school protects all of its students regardless of sexual orientation. This school doesn't need a special program or policy for that one group." Those of our schools that answer in this manner often do so because of community pressure to stay silent on issues related to sexual orientation.

Objections to the mention of sexual orientation in anti-bullying and anti-harassment policies results from fear that affirmation of our concern for LGBT students would indicate an acceptance of gays, lesbians, and bisexuals as a protected class of citizens and would give support to special rights for LGBT students. So rather than do this, we contend or pretend that our school protects LGBT students as it protects all of our students. Yet the data suggest that the schools that lack a clear statement of protection for LGBT students are also the schools that are likely to have higher incidence rates of harassment and attacks based on sexual orientation.[1] Sam, the boy in gym class who is perceived to be gay, is more likely to be bullied in the school where the policy is silent about sexual orientation than in the school that believes it important and necessary to mention these differences.

> In a survey conducted by Harris polling services, only 9 percent of principals felt that students were being harassed or bullied based on sexual orientation. In contrast, 28 percent of teachers and 34 percent of students reported seeing fellow students harassed or bullied based on sexual orientation (Harris Interactive 2008).

School principals are quick to recognize that bullying and harassment constitute a serious problem in the school setting. These administrators also tell us about the connection between being bullied or harassed and poor student performance. And they acknowledge that gay and lesbian students are more likely to be the brunt of harassment and bullying than are racial minorities, students with religious differences, or students with disabilities. Yet even when they recognize the increased vulnerability of LGB students, these principals still underestimate how often these students are harassed. In school the message is clear: bullying another student because of her or his race or religion will not be tolerated. The same is not true for taunts and jibes based on sexual orientation.

In a recent national survey, 60 percent of gay, lesbian, and bisexual students ages 13 to 21 reported feeling unsafe at school. Their sense of vulnerability was based on repeatedly witnessing and/or experiencing verbal harassment (86%), physical harassment (44%), and/or physical assaults (22%).[2] The feeling of fear was heightened when the homosexual or bisexual student felt that there were no consequences for the perpetrator.

Thirty-nine percent of students in this GLSEN (Gay, Lesbian, Straight Educators Network) survey reported that teachers or other staff members failed to intervene when they heard homophobic remarks. Sixteen percent of the students also reported that when they told administrators about instances of assault and harassment, these administrators took no action. These observations led students to feel even more vulnerable and to shy away from engaging with teachers and administrators. As we might guess, students enrolled in schools where anti-bullying policies included direct mention of sexual orientation were less likely to experience harassment and attacks.

> Richard, a student in the same junior high school I went to, was ostracized by most of his peers and ridiculed for his feminine behavior by at least one of his teachers. I don't know what his home life was like, but I do know that his school life wasn't too comfortable. When I heard he hung himself in his bedroom, I don't think I was surprised, but I was devastated—not just because Richard died in pain, but also because as a junior high school student, I wondered about what that meant about my own future. I was just beginning to understand that I was gay.

Being victimized by fellow students (experiencing direct harassment or bullying) and by staff (not being supported by administrators and teachers) can lead to consequences of varying degrees of severity. The fear of being the victim yet one more time may mean the choice of skipping or even dropping out of school. Living with fear will also affect learning—it's hard to study when you think you may be pummeled after school or when you experience depression. As destructive as dropping out of school may be, the consequences of classroom attacks can be worse.

Certainly not all LGB students are harassed or attacked. Many are never identified as homosexual or bisexual by peers. Others attend schools where it isn't "cool" to pick on someone because of sexual orientation (e.g., schools for performing arts). And increasing numbers of students in schools across the country are becoming accepting of these differences among peers. We also can't assume that every student who has negative experiences will drop out of school or have poor academic performance. Many will show great resilience, rising above the horrid experiences that shouldn't be happening in their lives, but are. But even with resilience and changes in attitudes, we need to ask ourselves whether schools should be allowed to ignore those students who do suffer under these all-too-common circumstances. And how do schools stop these events from happening?

On Tuesday, Feb. 12, 2008, an openly gay 8th grader named Lawrence King was shot to death by a classmate named Brandon McInerney at E.O. Green Junior High [located in Oxnard, California]. Brandon was threatened by Lawrence's self-acceptance of his sexual orientation and by his nontraditional gender expression, so threatened that he brought a gun to school and murdered Lawrence. . . . (a final and most extreme act in a pattern of bullying in which Brandon had engaged towards Lawrence for an extended period of time, a pattern which school officials seem to have done little to interrupt).

Oxnard's just up the 101 from Hollywood, less than an hour away from where *Will & Grace* and *Ellen* are filmed. I guess the students at E. O. Green Junior High just hadn't gotten the message that being LGBT is no big deal.

—Kosciw, Diaz, and Greytak 2008, vii

Few, if any, of us would support harassment or attacks on LGBT students. At the same time, there are numbers of us who oppose policies that provide for direct measures to stop or at least mitigate these incidences, fearing that having schools address these problems head-on would be yet one more step in approving homosexual behavior.[3] When we raise these objections, we are likely to offer one or some combination of three different arguments to justify our stance: (1) the problem of harassment and attacks is exaggerated, (2) the causes and supposed results of harassment and being attacked (depression, suicide) are in large part self-inflicted, and (3) explicitly protecting the safety of homosexual and bisexual students will take away from the rights of heterosexual students who dissent against same-sex behaviors.

The data on the severity of harassment of LGB students continues to point to an ongoing and serious problem. Almost one out of four LGB students reports being physically assaulted in the United States. A survey of teachers in England noted a similar trend. Rates of gay harassment and assaults on LGB students remain higher than attacks based on gender, disability, religion, or race.[4] With 25 percent of the students being physically harassed in high schools, it's difficult to claim that the problem is overstated, especially when these numbers are punctuated by suicides and the murders of individuals such as Lawrence King and Matthew Shepherd.

"If gay students didn't flaunt their sexual orientation, they wouldn't have so many problems." "When gay kids commit suicide or are unable to study

For several years, Jamie Nobozny was harassed and attacked in school because he was gay. These attacks included his classmates urinating on him and pretending to rape him. Once when he complained to school officials, they told him that as a gay male he had to expect harassment.

When he first sued the school district, a trial judge dismissed the case against the Ashland County Schools in Wisconsin. Upon appeal, a federal appellate court overturned the state court decision and found the district liable for close to $1 million (Lambda Legal 2009a).

because of depression, it demonstrates that they are mentally ill; mental illness is an unfortunate manifestation of being queer." These are two of the kinds of statements that support the idea that LGB students are the cause of their own problems.[5] The first of these statements suggests that if you act in a certain way, you can expect and possibly deserve to be attacked or harassed, an attitude not all that dissimilar from the idea that women who wear tight clothes can expect to be raped. "LGB students single themselves out for rejection and harassment. It is regrettable but predictable." Do we buy the same logic when we talk about the treatment of Jews throughout history, or the treatment of Christians in first-century Rome, or blacks in the Jim Crow South?

The second of the statements, which links homosexuality to inherent mental illness, ignores the findings of almost all mental health organizations. People who support these statements believe that depression, which may lead to poor school performance and tragic acts of suicide, is a manifestation of mental illness inherently associated with homosexuality: homosexuality = mental illness.

But for the vast majority of mental health professionals, the equation would be more accurately written,

homosexuality + rejection + derision = mental illness

or the following corollary equations:

homosexuality + rejection + derision + resiliency = success

homosexuality + acceptance = success

Where there is mental illness such as depression, the depression may well be a reaction to the bias and discrimination against homosexuality. In his book *The New Gay Teenager,* Savin-Williams points to the fact that LGB students are not inherently mentally ill and that even with society's negative responses, many LGB students fare quite well thanks to an inherent resiliency.

For many of us, the most interesting of the arguments raised in opposition to the direct mention of LGB students in anti-bullying policies is the assertion that such provisions will limit free speech for those students who object to same-sex behaviors. The case *Harper v. Poway* serves as a contemporary example where this argument has been played out in the courts.[6] In this case Poway High School's Gay–Straight Alliance held a day of silence protesting harassment and bias against homosexual students. On that day Tyler Chase Harper, a student at Poway, wore a t-shirt that had a statement on the front that read, "Be ashamed, our school embraced what God has condemned." The back of the shirt read, "I would die tonight for my beliefs." School administrators felt the shirt was derogatory and inflammatory. The school principle asked Harper to change shirts. Harper refused. Ruling on the ensuing freedom-of-speech lawsuit, the Ninth Circuit Court found that in the public school setting, administrators could and should censure speech if such speech is directed at a minority group and could cause those students harm (e.g., "Jews will burn in hell").

For those opposed to anti-bullying policies, *Harper v. Poway* demonstrated how provisions to protect LGB students would place limits on unfettered free speech by heterosexual peers who are committed to protecting society from homosexuality. Those who support provisions that would protect LGB students point to the fact that in public K–12 schools, we don't allow people of different religions to denigrate another religion (e.g., you couldn't wear a t-shirt that said "Devil Muslims Will Destroy American" or one that said "Christian Communion is Cannibalism"), nor do we allow students to make racially inflammatory statements (e.g. you can't wear t-shirts that suggest that God wants blacks to move back to Africa). The court ruled that although such actions can be accommodated in society in general, they should not occur in the school setting where minority or majority youth would be forced to confront these statements of denigration.

TO INCLUDE OR NOT INCLUDE—THAT IS THE QUESTION

To a naïve onlooker, it might seem that decisions to place a special focus of sexual orientation in anti-bullying policies should rest on the efficacy of such actions: Are there fewer assaults in schools that make specific mention of gay, lesbian, and bisexual students in these policies? Do LGB students feel safer in schools that include homosexual and bisexual students in their policy statements? But efficacy may be the last factor considered. Instead, other standards are used in making these types of decisions: local community mores, state and federal law, and professional and personal ethics. When all of these norms, including best practice, are in alignment, developing policy should be easy, but rarely do we find all of these norms lining up together.

Considering that schools can have heated conflicts when selecting math and reading curricula, it's easy to see why we have come to expect high levels of controversy when school districts consider including or intentionally excluding the mention of LGB students in their anti-bullying policies. Yet despite the controversy, a decision is inevitably reached—a decision that is often an attempt to avoid conflict.

What do our various standards say about this decision, and which of these standards do we use? Is it state or federal law that sets the practice? Is the school's first priority to safeguard community mores? Should school administrators follow their professional ethics? Do and should school systems rely on the personal beliefs of board members and chief administrators in making these choices? Or should schools follow best practices in protecting the safety of their students?

Legal Precedents

On issues related to anti-bullying policies, the legal landscape is much the same as the topography on workplace nondiscrimination—marked differences across jurisdictional lines. We have federal safe-school legislation and regulations, but within these rules there are no guiding principles covering this question.

This is not the case at the state level, where 38 states do have anti-bullying laws, 13 of which include specific mention of LGB students: California, Connecticut, Illinois, Iowa, Maine, Maryland, Massachusetts, Minnesota, New Jersey, Oregon, Vermont, Washington, and Wisconsin.[7] The other 25 state laws have no specific mention of LGB students. In some of the latter instances, there is no mention of any particular category (e.g., race, religion). The decision not to include any category is one way of circumventing the LGB student issue. Twelve states have no anti-harassment laws whatsoever on the books. In examining judicial action, we find court cases that insinuate protections must be provided if a school knows of harassment or attacks on LGB students, but these rulings require no preventive action.[8] This means that those school boards that don't have state mandates are free to act in any way they wish when putting together their anti-harassment provisions.

---

603 Commonwealth of Massachusetts Regulation, Section 26.07: Active Efforts:

(2) All public schools shall strive to prevent harassment or discrimination based upon students' race, color, sex, religion, national origin or sexual orientation, and all public schools shall respond promptly to such discrimination or harassment when they have knowledge of its occurrence.

—Massachusetts Department of Education 2001

Over the past few years an anti-bullying law has failed to pass in the North Carolina state legislature. One of the major reasons is that the bill's sponsor has insisted that the statute include sexual orientation in a list of characteristics specifically mentioned in the bill (Barge 2009).

Community Standards

Not unexpectedly, our state laws mirror our community standards. The majority of us do feel that schools have a responsibility for protecting our children against harassment and attacks from peers. And most of us would advocate for protecting homosexual and bisexual students from these behaviors. But there are many loud voices exhorting that this doesn't mean we should provide specific provisions for or accord special status to LGBT students. In these conversations we also hear those few voices that say if we want to protect LGBT students, let's say so unequivocally, lest silence be equated with an unspoken acceptance of harassment of these too often marginalized students. So we find two sets of community standards, and we are left to choose between what in many jurisdictions is the majority standard and the minority community standard.

Yes, homosexual students need to be protected from harm. But you don't want to encourage homosexuality. If you say no one should be harassed that should be enough. Listing gays in safe school policies is just one more part of the homosexual agenda.

—John, public school teacher

If it is not okay to say cocksucker, faggot, or lesbo make that prohibition as explicit as the prohibitions against the use of jungle bunny or nigger. We tell everyone that violence is not tolerated in schools, and then we spotlight race, gender or religion. Why don't we place the same emphasis on violence based on sexual orientation? When we don't do this it tells gays and lesbians to take cover.

—Terry, a college junior who was harassed while in high school

Professional Ethics

What of professional ethics—do they provide any guidelines for decisions on detailing sexual orientation? The nationally adopted ethics policies for the major K–12 professional groups provide no statements about specific school policies including harassment and anti-bullying, but each does offer precepts that provide guidance in deciding whether such policies should exist and whether to include sexual orientation in a given school's policies. The ethics policy for teachers, as defined by the National Education Association, calls on educators to protect students from exposure to harassment or disparagement. In the very next clause this policy prohibits discrimination against any student based on sexual orientation. It seems safe to assume that the first clause lends support to having anti-bullying policies. The second clause would suggest that if a failure to mention LGB students in a policy meant failure to provide the best protection for LGB students, teachers should be lobbying to include these students in the policy statement. School counselors have a set of similar statements in their code of ethics.[9]

In a contrast worth noting, the ethics policy for school administrators offers no provision for protecting the rights of specific groups of students. Nonetheless, this set of professional standards does have an interesting statement that obligates school administrators to "pursue appropriate measures to correct those laws, policies, and regulations that are not consistent with sound educational goals."[10] We might infer from this statement an ethical responsibility to challenge state laws and school policies that failed to protect gay, lesbian, and bisexual students.

Best Practice

The research documents a significant relationship between an explicit statement of protection for bisexual and homosexual students and (a) the number of reported incidents of LGB student harassment and (b) LGB students' perceived safety. In its most recent biennial study, GLSEN once again found that LGB students who attended schools with such policies experienced fewer occurrences of verbal harassment and physical attacks than their peers who attended schools with no anti-bullying policies or schools in which policies are silent about the needs of homosexual and bisexual students. Students attending proactive schools were also more likely to disclose such incidents to their teachers or school administrators, and authorities in these schools were more likely to intervene when these incidents were brought to their attention. In other words, silence about homosexuality is correlated with increased numbers of physical and verbal attacks.

> In order to make schools safe for all students and to prevent violence and harassment, schools should amend existing anti-harassment policies to include prohibiting violence, harassment, and verbal abuse directed against gay and lesbian students and those perceived to be gay or lesbian. Incidents of anti-gay abuse should be treated with the same discipline procedures as other incidents involving bias and hatred."
>
> —Massachusetts Department of Education 1995, no page

Reflecting on these survey outcomes, GLSEN makes a pointed call for school policies that directly speak to protection of bisexual and homosexual students:

One major step that schools can take to affirm their support for all students' safety is the implementation and enforcement of safe school policies. Safe school policies and laws can promote a better school climate for LGBT students when sexual orientation and/or gender identity/expression are explicitly addressed. GLSEN believes that the most effective policies are these types of comprehensive policies, those that explicitly provide protection by enumerating personal characteristics including sexual orientation and gender identity/expression.[11]

Despite the data collected in GLSEN's studies, a question that remains unanswered is whether the behaviors of the LGB students (greater likelihood of reporting incidents), their heterosexual peers (less likelihood of bullying LGB peers), and the teachers in these schools (acting on reports of harassment) are the direct result of the policy statement or are a manifestation of the school's social ecology. That is, schools that provide a safe space for LGB students also provide clear statements of policy reflecting the prevailing attitudes—which came first, the policy or the behavior?

But what we do know is that schools that refuse to openly state that they will protect gay, lesbian, and bisexual students are the schools where LGB students are most likely to encounter hostility and attacks from peers. When a school says, "We don't need to specify that we are talking about LGB students," it is identifying itself as an institution where this cohort of students will have the most difficulty. In cases like this, it might be time for school principals, teachers, and school counselors to consider their ethical principles.

THE SCHOOL'S SOCIAL ECOLOGY

If failure to change the school culture means more than 24,000 dropouts each year, along with 2,000 additional suicides or suicide attempts and another teen murdered, is the price too high? But what if changing the culture means an additional 50,000 high school students openly declaring their sexual orientation?

Policies on harassment are just one social convention that our educational institutions use to ensure the safety of LGB students, helping them to remain focused on their academics. The research also suggests that we build an ethos of belonging in which LGB students can openly express their sexual orientation and find positive role models standing in the front of the room and in the pages of the textbook.[12] If these changes in the social ecology of the schools are the steps we need to take to support the safety and academic success of homosexual and bisexual students, do we or do we not have an ethical imperative to build these characteristics into our schools?

Questions such as this inevitably bring us back to the same argument we have heard throughout many of the chapters in this text. Those of us seated on one side of the aisle see these proposed actions as yet one more attempt to normalize being gay—a step that will lead to the downfall of our civilization, including the destruction of our religious and social structures. Those of us gathered on the other side of the aisle see these actions as one more step toward normalizing being gay and a step that will open our society to an often oppressed and marginalized segment of our social community, leading to a more caring and just society. Both sides of the aisle believe that these actions will lead to homosexuality becoming more acceptable within society. Where we differ is how we measure the costs and benefits. While the argument rages on, some of us who are standing in the aisle are trying to avoid taking a seat while others are trying to decide which seat to take.

As we think about whether or not actions taken by K–12 schools will shift our societal views, we should acknowledge that most K–12 schools lag behind in reflecting changes in social mores, be they good or bad changes. All but the earliest adopters among schools tend to lag behind society, with late adopters at times appearing to be locked in a different century. Minus federal court decisions and laws, some K–12 schools would have taken a decade or more to begin desegregation. But schools will eventually catch up to the changes in society; it's just a matter of at what cost to the students who are in school today.

Those who think that the cost of inaction is too high propose some significant changes in the school culture—change that, as predicted by all, defines homosexuality and bisexuality as a normal part of the spectrum of human sexuality; change that allows students to openly acknowledge their sexual orientation without fear; change that allows LGB teachers and other staff members to do the same, serving as positive role models in and outside the classroom; change that supports student organizations such as the gay–straight alliances that are appearing on more and more high school campuses; and change that recognizes and supports full participation by same-sex couples who have children enrolled in the school.

Any change in ecology that allows LGB students to come out of the closet; opens the school doors to gay, lesbian, and bisexual teachers; and opens the parent–teacher association to same-sex couples who are raising straight children will inevitably offend some. When we help calm the fears of the parents who accept their child's sexual orientation but are concerned about how their child will be received in the classroom, we alienate parents who are having a difficult time accepting their daughters or sons' homosexual desires.

Several years ago, a student in one of my graduate courses asked if she could meet with me after class. She proceeded to tell me the story of her 11-year-old son, who was being bullied at school. Early in the conversation, she told me that she was reasonably certain he was gay but that he hadn't realized it himself yet—it was still too early in his development to think about his own sexuality. According to her, when she took the matter to the school, they pretty well washed their hands of any responsibility. She and her husband were fine with the fact that their son might be gay; her brother was, and both she and her husband loved that brother. But she didn't want her son punished at school for a characteristic that was in his genetic code (her words). A month ago, I ran into a young girl who was living through quite a different experience. Her mother and father had recently found text messages from her girlfriend. The text messages made it apparent that they were beginning to date. With this revelation and after consulting with someone at their church, Mom and Dad had taken away the cell phone, put their daughter on restrictions, and started to throw out her all-too-masculine wardrobe.

> In building the case for same-sex marriage in Iowa, Jen and Dawn Bo-browski tell the story of trying to find the right preschool for one of their daughters. When looking at one school they asked if there would be any problems because their daughter came from a two-mother home. The director said no, but of course the young girl wouldn't be allowed to share the fact that she had two mothers when it came time to describe her family life (Taylor 2009).

These different sets of parents are going to want very different things from their local school system. If we create a welcoming and supportive environment, we meet the expectations of the mother with the 11-year-old son; if we are silent (e.g., no mention of homosexuality in our anti-bullying policy) or negative (not allowing students to start a gay–straight alliance) on issues related to homosexuality, we meet the expectations of the parents with the daughter who is coming out but leave the 11-year-old unprotected. The question we have to ask ourselves is, which norms do we follow: best practices, professional ethics, prevailing community standards? We might also ask ourselves these questions: What does the child need from the school? And how do we accommodate those needs as best we can? These certainly aren't easy questions to answer, but they are real questions that schools are answering every day, and with every answer someone is offended. And with some answers, our children are harmed, sometimes irreparably.

THE FORMAL CURRICULUM

One of the more controversial elements in the effort to change the social ecology in K–12 schools is the call to modify the curriculum. The argument most frequently offered in support of these modifications is that all students have a right to see themselves in their textbooks, discovering the roles that individuals like them have played throughout history. A second and possibly more compelling argument is that failure to include and acknowledge homosexual and bisexual persons and related issues in the curriculum is a conscious distortion of fact—government-sanctioned propaganda by censorship. A third argument is that by including LGB people and issues in the curriculum, we can help inform the ongoing cultural debates. Each of these arguments recognizes that what is ignored can be every bit as important as what is included in our curricula.

And Tango Makes Three is a beautifully illustrated children's book that tells the story of Roy and Silo, two male chinstrap penguins who lived in the Central Park Zoo and hatched an egg, nurturing Tango, a female chick, into penguin adulthood. With an elegantly written narrative by Peter Parnell and Justin Richardson (2005), this national award–winning text helps children understand that families come in various forms and flavors. It has become a lightning rod for the anger felt by those who oppose and fear these various curricular changes. For those of us who were denied the right to know that many of our favorite authors and composers as well as many of our heroes and heroines were just like us, *And Tango Makes Three* is an example of what school could have been like.

When something is included in the curriculum, it tells the student that society considers it important. But when we leave material out of our books and class discussions, we telegraph other messages—the material may not be important or valued; the material may be something we hide in polite society. Our children know that homosexuality exists; they learn this on the playground at recess and on the bus ride home. When it's not talked about in the classroom or at home, the message is that it must be something that should be hidden. This is especially true if and when our children begin to recognize these types of feelings inside themselves. Silence is in no way neutral ground. Silence is loud and indisputable disapproval.

Recognizing the strong objections from those who believe that proposed changes to the curriculum are a thinly veiled attempt to recruit more children into homosexuality, those of us who support these changes hope that a more honest curriculum will allow homosexual and bisexual children to understand that they are a worthy and integral part of society. We also want children raised by same-sex parents to feel welcome and respected in the classroom. And finally, we want open and informed dialogue in the society.

At the elementary school level, two learning outcomes that are commonly identified include (1) acceptance and respect for difference and (2) awareness that human families come in all different forms, including some with same-sex parents. The modifications commonly recommended at the secondary level begin with (1) acknowledging the sexual orientation of key historic and literary figures, allowing students to see these figures as role models, and (2) discussion of events such as the Stonewall riots in social studies classes, allowing students to understand their history (see chapter 6, "The Downfall of Society," in this text). There is also a call to include sexual orientation in human sexuality courses and to acknowledge that homosexual and bisexual behaviors occur across species in biology classes. At the collegiate level, queer or gay studies courses should be available, much like our gender and black studies courses.[13] As we propose these changes, we must also understand that the curriculum must be open to voices that oppose rights for gay men, lesbians, and bisexuals and that the many historic opponents of these rights should also be a part of the curriculum. Our discussions from either side of the aisle must be civil and respectful when they occur in the classroom.

When we talk about including recognition of sexual orientation and homosexual issues in the curriculum, we are opening ourselves to a maelstrom of criticism. The intelligent design–versus–evolution debate may seem like a child's party compared to the battles we will have when we mention that Tennessee Williams was gay while students read his plays or that Michelangelo was homosexual while students view slides of the Sistine Chapel. And just wait for the discussion in biology class about the members of different species who don't reproduce because they prefer relationships with same-sex mates. Some may wonder, why on earth would we mention any of this? One good reason would be because it's true, and we don't lie by commission or omission. A second good reason would be so that when those of us who are gay or lesbian sit in the classroom, we understand that we are a part of nature's design and that we too can write the great American novel, create the next great economic theory, serve in the Congress of the United States, win an Olympic Gold Medal, or win a Nobel Prize. We also have a right to expect that the heterosexual student sitting next to us understands that we have no reason to hide who we are. No doubt, having students learn about evolution is important and in keeping with our responsibility to educate students honestly and openly, but having them learn about homosexuality will have more practical impact in the course of their day-to-day lives, despite the storm that it will unleash.

STRAIGHT ANSWERS

All students deserve to be safe and protected in the school setting. This is about as close to a universally accepted principle in education as we are going to find. Regrettably, however, data on schoolyard harassment tell us that not all students are protected, with lesbian, gay, and bisexual students being among the most vulnerable. And the price the unprotected student pays can be devastating and at times even fatal.

When we look for answers as to why and where LGB students are at greater risk, we discover that these particular students are safer in schools that adopt anti-bullying policies that expressly forbid harassing or attacking homosexual or bisexual students. We don't know whether this is because of the policies themselves or the result of the general attitudes and standards in schools that have the fortitude to adopt these policies. That is, these schools take student safety seriously and are cognizant of the particular needs of LGBT students. What we do know is that those schools that remain silent on protection of LGBT students fail to protect gay, lesbian, bisexual, and transgender students as effectively as their sister institutions. Recognizing this, we need to make clear that the statement "Our school doesn't single out homosexual students because we protect all students" really means "Our school is uncomfortable with addressing the issue" or "Our school has a bias against gay, lesbian, bisexual, and transgender students."

If we intend to protect LGBT students, we need to make explicit our commitment, and we must support that commitment with action. Silence and inaction don't work. At the very least, every gay, lesbian, bisexual, or transgender student must know that any staff member will stop harassment when the staff member sees it. And if the student reports an incident to any adult in the school, the student will be treated with respect and care, and the allegation will be examined. If the allegation is proven to be true, there will be consequences for the perpetrator. This should be the minimum threshold, with schools and professionals that fail to meet this standard subject to prosecution.

Meeting the basic need for safety is a good start, but it is only a start. To address dropout rates among LGBT students, we need to reconstruct schools, replacing hostility with affirmation. And if we want to equip LGBT students with the information they will need to understand themselves and the world in which they live, we must replace the censorship of silence with open and honest discussion. The courts and federal law have been explicit about telling schools that they need to allow gay–straight student clubs.[14] Nonetheless, there are schools that continually try to shut these support groups down by saying no when students begin to organize these alliances or by putting up roadblocks to membership. The messages that are being sent to the LGBT students are "You and your kind are not welcome in this school" and "We really don't care if you drop out"—the same messages echoed by the textbook censorship.

Thirty years ago, almost no one talked about homosexuality in the public forum, but since 1969 and the Stonewall Riots, that has been changing. Since then the American Psychiatric Association, the American Bar Association, the American Pediatric Association, and the National Education Association have all said we must stop the persecution. And today homosexuality is a topic of conversation in which we all engage regularly. So why do our public schools continue to remain silent? Certainly it's not because we think that students are unaware of the ongoing dialogue or that schools have a responsibility to shield students. Schools remain silent for one of two reasons—they equate silence with neutrality, or they recognize that with the shift in cultural and professional standards, they have lost the ability to condemn homosexuality openly, so they say nothing and condemn by silence. Neither of these reasons paints a particularly affirming or positive picture of the school boards or the professionals who run America's public schools, especially when we consider the fact that their silence, for whatever reason, continues to equate with more dropouts and suicides as well as ongoing cultural illiteracy. This is not the hallmark of the educational system we ought to have in this the land of the free and home of the brave. But alas, it is, at least for now, where we are.

NOTES

1. Harris Interactive 2005.
2. Kosciw, Diaz, and Greytak 2008.

3. Cloud 2005.

4. Kosciw, Diaz, and Greytak 2008; Winterman 2008.

5. Lipkin 2003.

6. Mercurio and Morse 2007.

7. Family Equality Council 2008.

8. Lambda Legal 2009a; Mercurio and Morse 2007.

9. American School Counselor Association 2006; National Education Association 1975; Satcher and Leggett 2007.

10. American Association of School Administrators 2007.

11. Harris 2008, p. xvi.

12. Harris 2008; Savin-Williams 2005.

13. Serwatka and Carroll 1999.

14. American Civil Liberties Union 2007; Lambda Legal Defense Fund 2009b.

10

Straight Talk

Throughout these pages we have been looking at the ongoing debates on homosexuality and bisexuality, asking a number of explicit and implicit queer questions arising from these debates. In some instances we have discovered very definitive answers; in other cases our hypotheses are tentative and incomplete, awaiting a great deal more research before we can lock in the final answer. And for some of our questions, we have multiple and differing answers with which we will need to live (You say tə-mā'-tō; I say tə-mä'-tō), despite our desire to cast everything in red or blue or right or wrong.

In chapter 6, we asked whether the Roman Empire and Ancient Greece fell because they openly accepted these varied expressions of human sexuality. History tells us that the answer to this question is a straightforward and simple *no*. It's clear that homosexuality and bisexuality can be seen across time and, most probably, throughout all civilizations. History also tells us that these variances in sexual orientation have been openly accepted in several of the most successful civilizations that have existed on this planet. The reality is that the often-mentioned relationships between homosexuality and the fall of the Greek and Roman civilizations are nothing more than badly distorted history. Instead, what we find is that the most repressive of societies have been among the most hostile to homosexuals and bisexuals. However, the reverse has not always been true; not all societies that have been open and accepting of same-sex love have also been void of repression.

In chapters 8 and 9, we discussed whether there is there a secret homosexual agenda. No doubt about it, there is a move to secure civil and economic rights for lesbians, gay men, and bisexuals, but it is far from secret. In fact, it is rather well advertised. Whether or not you place the name *agenda* on this movement is really personal choice. But these efforts—agenda or human rights movement—do not extend to advocating for polygamy or lowering the age of consent any more than conservative Christianity advocates for separation of the races. Some few voices in both these movements have taken and still take these extreme positions, but the vast majority of women and men in these movements certainly don't. Raising these issues is one of the scare tactics used by the most frightened and the most calculating of the opponents to LGBT rights. This human rights movement also doesn't ask for special status (i.e., affirmative action) for LGBT individuals. Nor does this agenda call for quotas. It does, however, include some highly controversial elements, including same-sex marriage and opening the curriculum in public K–12 schools and colleges.

On several occasions we have arrived at more tentative answers. In answering the question asked in chapter 2—how many homosexuals and bisexuals are there?—we find no solid evidence that would support the often-promoted idea that 10 percent of the population is homosexual. Setting aside Kinsey's questionable data, we do have data from a number of national and international studies that suggest that at least 4 to 6 percent of males are either homo- or bisexual and at least 2 to 4 percent of females are either homo- or bisexual. In looking at these data over time, we find an ongoing trend in which greater numbers of people are reporting themselves as belonging to one of these categories. I assume this trend results from the growing social acceptance of differing sexual orientations; with this greater acceptance comes an increasing willingness to come out of the closet. This gives us reason to believe that actual percentages may be higher than so far reported, but we will need more time, more definitive measures, and better ways to collect our data to make any such judgment.

Whatever the final answer, we need to consider whether the number of LGB individuals should be the basis for granting or denying human rights. Do you get your rights only if you are 10 percent of the population? If so, Jews, redheads, deaf people, blind people, and a whole lot of other groups are fair game for discrimination.

Our answer to what the origins of homosexuality are also remains somewhat up in the air. In chapter 3, we discussed an expanding and compelling body of research that links sexual orientation to biological origins. This literature documents same-sex couplings throughout the animal kingdom. In some species this means an individual animal moves back and forth between same-sex coupling and opposite-sex encounters. For other animals this means a lifelong attraction to members of the same sex. There is a solid body of research pointing to genetic and other biochemical triggers in humans. But this research has not uncovered *the* gay gene, nor is it likely to do so. As with many biologically influenced traits, the puzzle is much more complicated than that. But the data do offer a high degree of certainty that biology provides at least one determinant—one or more genetic elements—and very probably a second set of determinants, hormones. When we finally have an answer, it seems certain that environment will also play a role, which may be limited to how we express sexual orientation in a given society. But changing the way we parent isn't going to give us more or fewer homosexuals and bisexuals. However, it will mean the difference between well-adjusted and less-well-adjusted homosexuals and bisexuals.

Chapter 5 focused on the question of whether gay men and lesbians can convert to heterosexuality. Data from different sources causes us to be very skeptical about how often such conversions occur and how effective these conversions really are. First, Spitzer's study, which purports to have proven that these therapies work, was poorly designed, and even after months of working with reparative therapists from across the nation, he still was unable to locate a sufficient number of men and women who would state that their sexual orientation had changed. In Erzen's ethnographic study on church-based reparative therapy, we discover that few men and fewer women show up for these therapeutic programs. And of those that do, most leave before completing the programs, dropping out frustrated by their lack of progress or their inability to control their sexual desires. Those who complete these programs tell us that being an ex-gay isn't the same thing as being a born-again heterosexual; you don't develop the same kinds of attractions to women or to men, although some men and women may develop a relationship of sorts.

Coupled with the anecdotal stories of failure, these bits of research provide good reason to believe that reparative therapy falls far short of the claims raised in the 1998 public relations campaign and that advocates of reparative therapy have failed to come forward with any objective literature to argue otherwise. Haldeman offers what is probably the most cogent suggestion for therapists working with lesbians and gay men who are uncomfortable with their sexual orientation because of religious conflict. Haldeman suggests that the therapist begin by helping the individual accept his or her sexual orientation. Once there is acceptance, work with the individual to find a path for reconciling the person's religious conviction with his or her acknowledged sexual orientation. This may take the form of celibacy with open acknowledgment of homosexuality, or it could mean finding a religious faith that welcomes lesbians and gay men into the fold. Or for those who are bisexual, it could take the form of establishing a committed heterosexual relationship, recognizing that there will be homosexual attractions throughout life but that these don't need to be acted on. Whichever path the therapy follows, it needs to be based on complete honesty, and it needs to be the path the client selects, without prejudice or pressure from the therapist.

For some of our questions, we found that there are really multiple correct answers and few if any incorrect answers. When we asked whether sacred scripture condemns homosexuality, we discovered that the answer depends on who is interpreting the religious text. If we don't believe in the particular scriptures, the question of what the sacred texts say is without merit or consequence to us. This rejection of whole bodies of scriptures or different elements within scriptures is certainly not unique to the discussion of homosexuality or to our times. Jews don't accept the New Testament; Christians don't accept the Qur'an. For Thomas Jefferson the teachings of Christ served as a compelling moral and ethical code, but he rejected those passages in the Bible that spoke of miracles and the divinity of Jesus. This is similar to Mohamed's understanding of the New Testament; Christ was a prophet but not a God. Similarly, for today's mainstream and fundamentalist Christians, whole sections of the Old Testament, including those that deal with dietary laws, are put aside as irrelevant to today's culture.

If we have a set of scripture that we do accept, we must then determine how the passages should have been translated and then how the translation should be interpreted. For those of us who are nonbelievers, Sodom and Gomorrah is an interesting myth. But for all of us who believe that it is a factually based story of God's intervention or an inspired allegory, we still need to determine which interpretation of the story we believe. Some of us may go back to interpretations that were offered at the time Jesus walked the earth—the people of Sodom and Gomorrah had forsaken God's law to treat strangers with love and care and were punished for their callous treatment of others, which they demonstrated by an attempted rape of God's angels. For those of us who accept the interpretation first introduced by Josephus 60-some years after Jesus died, the sin is, at least in part, tied to homosexuality. In a pluralistic society each of these interpretations ought to be permissible, just as are our different interpretations of whether the universe was literally created in six days or the wine and bread become the actual blood and body in the Eucharist.

There are also multiple answers to the question asked in chapter 7: what do gay men and lesbians look like? Those of us who are gay look and act like human beings—some of us are very colorful, but more of us are very plain and ordinary. Some of us are terribly flawed, some are saint-like, and most of us fall somewhere in between. Some of us are easily identified as being gay; others are known only when we choose to disclose our sexual orientation (i.e., out ourselves). Most of us have the inevitable emotional problems that come with being human; others of us have additional problems that are exacerbated by societal and familial rejection. We are the everyman and everywoman, and we are the Nobel Prize winner and the artist whose work is admired for centuries and even millennia.

As we find the answers to our questions, we inevitably find even more questions—a frustration and gift for the human mind. Personally, I want things neat and orderly; it makes everything so easy to organize. But then what would I do with my God-given talents to assess, balance, nuance, and value?

How do we balance the research that indicates women are more fluid in their sexual orientation than their male counterparts against the research that demonstrates that genetics plays a more significant role in women's sexual orientation? Why are women more likely to move from heterosexual to homosexual behaviors (e.g., the mothers of four of my closest friends) and from homosexual to heterosexual relationships (e.g., apparently Ann Hecht the actress) than are men,[1] who are less likely to shift identity once they have become comfortable with having sex with other men?

What leads to the fact that some LGB youth flourish despite a hostile atmosphere at home and in school, whereas others are driven to depression and even suicide by the taunts and jeers they hear from parent and peer? What leads to victimization versus resiliency in these situations?

How do we assess which society exerts more influence on the expressions of same-sex love? Does an open and welcoming society shape the behavior more, or does a hostile culture have more influence, even though the behaviors shaped in this society are less healthy? Is it better to encourage open acknowledgement and self-acceptance, or do we want to encourage hiding in the shadows?

RECURRING THEMES

In exploring the answers to the questions that underlie the current gay debates, we keep running into recurring themes: the battle between good and evil; the continual retelling of the same stories to support one or the other perspective, even when these stories are outdated or flat-out wrong; expressions of the distrust of difference; and arguments over whose liberties we protect and at what cost to the other person. "Homosexuals want to destroy our society" versus "Heterosexuals are working to keep us as second-class or marginalized citizens." "Gay men are trying to legalize sex with underage children" versus "Antigay forces are using shock therapy in their failed attempts to change sexual orientation." "I should not be able to be fired just because I am homosexual" versus "I should not lose my right to free speech and the free expression of my religion just because of a corporate nondiscrimination policy." These themes aren't all that different from the themes we see throughout many of our political campaigns and much of our public discourse. When we are engaged in conflict, we tend to adopt these same strategies on both sides of the aisle. Of course, in these instances we have a proclivity to recognize the wrongheadedness of these behaviors when they occur on the other side.

We also have seen how those of us who are on opposite sides of the aisle can take the same data and come to very different conclusions. For some of us, a higher rate of suicide among homosexual teenagers leads us to believe that homosexual teenagers are at greater risk of developing profound depression because of the way they're treated by family and the world around them. On the other side of the aisle, these data demonstrate that homosexual teenagers are inherently mentally ill; it is just part of the syndrome. For some of us, the research that supports a biological link demonstrates that differing sexual orientations are a part of nature; for others of us, this research may tell us how much like animals homosexuals are or that we will someday find the cure for the disease.

These recurring themes and the strident voices we hear on both sides of the conflict are a clear signal of how high the stakes are in our disagreements over homosexuality. Many of us who are lesbian, gay, or bisexual see these conflicts as an immediate and ongoing threat to our personal dignity and to our survival—a denial of life, liberty, and the pursuit of happiness. We also carry with us a sense of responsibility to protect those who are following behind us, to build a world that will treat gay, lesbian, and bisexual youth more humanely than it has treated us. We are in some ways their surrogate parents. At other times we may be acting out of anger—an anger arising from the dreams denied and the all-too-real pains inflicted.

For those who oppose LGB rights, these conflicts are as much a war for society's soul as they are a battle over same-sex expressions of love. We are convinced that without asserting our will over others, the world will surely fall apart. This is not just about gay and lesbian rights; it is about control over the destiny of the human race. After all, haven't we heard our religious and social leaders link these sinful behaviors to pedophilia, disease, and the crumbling of the American family? In our battle against the not-so-secret homosexual agenda, we must question anyone who opposes us on this and any other issue. If that political candidate supports same-sex marriage, she has failed the litmus test and must be defeated, or she may lead us down the all-too-slippery road.

These battles also help bind us together. If we want to get more conservatives to the polls, just put an anti-gay initiative on the ballot in a red state. If we are a liberal lobbying group in need of funding, just find an outside threat to rally our troops.

Although the answers to the questions we have asked throughout the book can help inform our debates, the answers certainly won't stop these battles. But we can use our answers to jettison some of the recurring slogans and sound bites that are simply wrong, taking a small step forward in our discussions: homosexuality was not the cause of the downfall of Rome, and Kinsey did not prove that 10 percent of the population is homosexual. If after leaving behind these bad pieces of folklore, we can then come to agreement about collecting the missing pieces of information, we would take an even larger step in the right direction: let's use the U.S. census to begin collecting the data on same-sex relationships, and if we believe reparative therapy works, let's do some honest research tracking the men and women who enter and leave these programs.

Regrettably, discarding patently false accusations and assertions and conducting honest data collection cause us to fear that we will lose control, and that's why we passionately avoid these actions—"I need to shout, if I am to be heard over their shouting." "I can't open up to complete scrutiny before I know what the answer is going to be. It might weaken my position." We also understandably have a fear of waiting too long—"How long do I need to wait to be treated as a full member of society?" "How many teenagers must be subjected to rejection and ridicule?" "How much longer can society survive this spiral into immorality?"

In many ways these recurring themes and our fears over ceding control may lead these battles to continue for what seems like an eternity. After all, haven't Jews and Christians been fighting for over 2,000 years, and haven't Arabs, Christians, and Jews been fighting for the last 1,400 years? And there is no promise that the conflicts will stop soon.

Yet history does offer us some hope, along with clear notes of caution. If we examine the struggles for gender and race equity, we can see how historic change can and does occur—a woman and a black man running against each other to represent the political party that was destined to win the 2008 U.S. presidential election is no small step. And if we track the current polls, we find significant shifts in attitudes about human rights for gay men, lesbians, and bisexuals. But when we search history, we also come across major reversals of fortune. In the early 1900s there was an emerging movement to secure equal rights for homosexuals in Germany and other parts of Europe. In the same time frame, there was a growing body of research on the origins of homosexuality and an increasingly more accepting atmosphere in major cities such as Berlin. In the mid-1930s, with the rise of the Third Reich, all of this came tumbling down. The books were burned, the research was stopped, hundreds of thousands of homosexuals went back into the closet, and tens of thousands were sent to their death in concentration camps.

In America we speak of life, liberty, and the pursuit of happiness as inalienable rights—rights that cannot be denied or given away. Securing these rights has been an uphill fight for many and should not be taken for granted by any. But securing or maintaining my rights does not require or allow me to deny someone else his rights. In fact, the only way my rights can be secure is if I recognize the rights of others to dissent from and differ with me. I must work to ensure that Brother Isaiah, an itinerant preacher who comes to our campus once or twice a year, retains his right to yell at every passerby about her or his sins—"faggot," "whore," "baby killer," "Jesus killer," "Pope worshipper," "drunkard"—even when I am offended by his profanity and his attacks. But Brother Isaiah needs to understand that his freedom of speech and religion cannot abridge my freedom to love the man in my life, the man who challenges me to become a better and more committed person, the man who kneels beside me at the communion rail, the man who makes me laugh and holds me when I cry. Nor can Brother Isaiah's right to explore his beliefs be used to abridge my rights to learn what science and history have to tell me about myself and what pains those who have come before me have suffered and what they have done to enrich this world. If Brother Isaiah believed the world was flat, would that mean I couldn't study the science that paints quite a different picture? Brother Isaiah, shoot your verbal arrows if you so choose, but allow me to live in liberty, pursuing happiness by expressing the love my creator has given to me.

In many ways my own family serves as an example of this standard of behavior. Some members of my family have embraced and celebrate my homosexuality, whereas others continue to see it as a sin against God and question my judgment in being open about my sexual orientation. But all of them have come to understand that this is who I am, and if they want me in their lives, they have to accept me as I am, with life partner in tow.

It would bring me great joy if all of my family came to rejoice in this part of my given nature or if they would at least make an honest effort to study the issues from both sides before they draw their conclusions, but I love them no matter what their beliefs on this topic and appreciate their unquestioned love for me and their understanding that it is my life to live with the values I hold dear. Some family members have changed their understanding of homosexuality, and others have not, and we have had our battles over this topic, but none of them see me as a threat to their marriages or to their children. I am the son, the brother, the uncle that God and nature gave to them, and they are among some of the most precious gifts that I have received.

My efforts to understand who I am will continue until I die, but I feel better informed and at greater peace having taken the time to study this part of my being. Dad, thank you for giving me tools I needed to follow this path. I am a lucky man to have had you and Mom as parents.

NOTE

1. Diamond 2003, 2007.

APPENDIX

Reported Incidences of Same-Sex Behavior in Adulthood, Same-Sex Attraction, and Homosexual and Bisexual Self-Identity

Population studied Researchers/reference	Number of respondents		Percent reporting same-sex attraction		Percent reporting same-sex behaviors in adulthood		Percent self-identifying as homosexual or bisexual	
	Male	Female	Male	Female	Male	Female	Male	Female
U.S. Laumann, Gagnon, Michael, and Michaels 1994	3,917	4,827	3.7%[a]	1.7%[a]	6.4%[b]	3.5%[b]	2.8%	1.4%
Australia and New Zealand Smith, Rissel, Richters, Grulich, and de Visser 2003	10,173	9,134	2.3%[c]	1.8%[c]	2.0%[b]	1.0%[b]	2.5%	2.2%
Britain in 1990 Wellings, Wadsworth, and Johnson 1994	8,335	10,412	1.5%[a]	0.7%[a]	3.7%[b]	1.9%[b]	n/a	n/a
Britain in 2000 Erens, McManus, Prescott, and Field 2001	3,392	4,747	2.4%[c]	1.4%[c]	6.3%[b]	5.7%[b]	n/a	n/a
			Reporting same-sex behavior and/or attraction		Reporting same-sex behavior			
U.S., Britain, and France Sell, Wells, and Wypij 1995 U.S.	1,288	634	20.8%[d]	17.8%[d]	6.2%[e]	3.6%[e]	n/a	n/a
UK	1,137	696	16.3%[d]	18.6%[d]	4.5%[e]	2.1%[e]	n/a	n/a
France	1,506	788	18.5%[d]	18.5%[d]	10.7%[e]	3.3%[e]	n/a	n/a

[a]Desire, attraction or appeal to same gender.
[b]Having at least one same-gender partner within past five years.
[c]An equal, predominant, or exclusive attraction to same gender.
[d]Attraction to or sexual behavior with same-gender partner in the past five years.
[e]At least one homosexual experience in the past five years.

Bibliography

Acs, G., and S. Neslon. 2003. *Changes in family structure and child well-being: Evidence from the 2002 national survey of America's families.* Washington, D.C.: The Urban Institute. http://www.urban.org/UploadedPDF/311025_family_ structure.pdf.

Adams, H. E., L. W. Wright, and B. A. Lohr. 1996. "Is homophobia associated with homosexual arousal?" *Journal of Abnormal Psychology* 105: 440–45.

Ailey, S. H., B. A. Marks, C. Crisp, and J. E. Hahn. 2003. "Promoting sexuality across the life span for individuals with intellectual and developmental disabilities." *The Nursing Clinics of North America: Intellectual and Developmental Disabilities* 38: 227–49.

Aldrich, R. 2006. "Gay and lesbian history." In *Gay life and culture: A world history,* ed. R. Aldrich, pp. 7–28. London: Thames & Hudson.

Alyson. 1993. "People." In *The Alyson almanac 1994–1995 edition: The fact book of the lesbian and gay community,* pp. 118–202. Boston: Author.

American Association of School Administrators. 2007. *AASA's statement of ethics for educational leaders.* http://www.aasa.org/content.aspx?id=1390.

American Civil Liberties Union. 2007. *Federal judge rules Okeechobee, Florida, students can form gay-straight alliance club.* http://www.aclu.org/lgbt/youth/ 29283prs20070406.html.

American Psychiatric Association. 1998. *Position statement on psychiatric treatment and sexual orientation.* Arlington, VA: Author.

American Psychiatric Association. 2000. *Therapies focused on attempts to change sexual orientation (reparative or conversion therapies).* Arlington, VA: Author.

American Psychological Association. 2006. *Guideline for psychotherapy with lesbian, gay, & bisexual clients.* Washington, D.C.: Author.

American School Counselor Association. 2006. *Ethical standards for school counselors.* Alexandria, VA: Author.

Andersen, R., and T. Fetner. 2008. "Cohort differences in tolerance of homosexuality: Attitudinal change in Canada and the United States, 1981–2000." *Public Opinion Quarterly* 72: 311–30.

Aquinas, Saint Thomas. 1952. *The summa theological: Vol. II.* Trans. the Fathers of the English Dominican Province. Chicago: William Benton.

Augustine, Saint. 1952. *The confessions of the city of God on Christian doctrine.* Trans. Edward Bouverie Pusey. Chicago: William Benton.

Austin, B. S. n.d. *Homosexuals and the Holocaust.* http://frank.mtsu.edu/~baustin/homobg.html.

Avery, A., J. Chase, L. Johansson, S. Litvak, D. Montero, and M. Wydra. 2007. "America's changing attitudes toward homosexuality, civil unions and same-gender marriage." *Social Work* 52(1): 71–80.

Bagemihl, B. 1999. *Biological exuberance: Animal homosexuality and natural diversity.* New York: St. Martin's Press.

Bailey, D. S. 1995. *Homosexuality and the western Christian tradition.* Hamden, CT: Archon Books.

Bailey, J. M., D. Bobrow, M. Wolfe, and S. Mikach. 1995. "Sexual orientation of adult children of gay fathers." *Developmental Psychology* 31: 124–29.

Bailey, J. M., and M. Oberschneider. 1997. "Sexual orientation and professional dance." *Archives of Sexual Behavior* 26: 433–42.

Bailey, J. M., and R. C. Pillard. 1991. "A genetic study of male sexual orientation." *Archives of Genetic Psychology* 48: 1089–96.

Bailey, J. M., R. C. Pillard, M. C. Neale, and Y. Agyei. 1993. "Heritable factors influencing sexual orientation in women." *Archives of Genetic Psychology* 50: 277–93.

Baines, J. 1985. "Egyptian twins." *Orientalia* 54: 461–82.

Baldwin, J. D., and J. I. Baldwin. 1989. "The socialization of homosexuality and heterosexuality in a non-western society." *Archives of Sexual Behavior* 18: 13–29.

Bancroft, J. 2003. "Can sexual orientation change? A long running saga." *Archives of Sexual Behavior* 32: 419–23.

Barge, J. M. 2009. "Equality NC kicks of 2009 with renewed efforts to pass school violence prevention act." Out in the Carolinas Publishing. http://www.stereotypd.com/index.php/component/content/article/137-equality-nc-kicks-off-2009-with-renewed-effort-to-pass-school-violence-prevention-act.html.

Bartos, L., and J. Holeckova. 2006. "Exciting ungulates: male-male mounting in fallow, white-tailed and red deer." In *Homosexual behaviour in animals: An evolutionary perspective,* ed. V. Sommer and P. L. Vasey, pp. 154–71. Cambridge: Cambridge University Press.

Battle, J., and A. J. Lemelle. 2002. "Gender differences in African American attitudes toward gay males." *The Western Journal of Black Studies* 26: 134–39.

Bawer, B. 1994. *A place at the table: The gay individual in American society.* New York: Touchstone Books.

Bayer, R. 1987. *Homosexuality and American psychiatry.* Princeton: Princeton University Press.

BBC News. 2006. "Afghan on trial for Christianity." March 20. http://news.bbc.co.uk/2/hi/south_asia/4823874.stm.

Beck, G. 1999. *An underground life: Memoirs of a gay Jew in Nazi Germany.* Madison: The University of Wisconsin Press.

Bennett, L., and G.J. Gates. 2004. *The cost of marriage inequity to children and their same-sex parents.* Washington, D.C.: Human Rights Campaign.

Bensen, W.R. 2003. *Anything but straight: Unmasking the scandals and lies behind the ex-gay myth.* New York: Harrington Park Press.

Benstock, S. 1989. "Paris lesbianism and the politics of reaction: 1900–1940." In *Hidden from history: Reclaiming the gay and lesbian past,* ed. M.B. Duberman, M. Vicinus, and G. Chauncey, pp. 332–46. New York: New American Library.

Bensyl, D.M., A.D. Iuliani, M. Carter, J. Santelli, and B.C. Gilbert. 2005. "Contraceptive use—United States and territories, behavioral risk factor surveillance system (2002)." *MMWR Surveillance Summaries* 54(18): 1–72.

Berglund, H., P. Lindström, and I. Savic. 2006. "Brain response to putative pheromones in lesbian women." *Proceedings of the National Academy of Sciences of the United States of America* 103: 8269–74.

Bernstein, R.A. 2003. *Straight parents, gay children: Keeping families together.* New York: Thunder's Mouth Press.

Bickham, P.J., S.L. O'Keefe, E. Baker, G. Berhie, M.J. Kommor, and K.V. Harper-Dorton. 2007. "Correlates of early overt and covert sexual behaviors in heterosexual women." *Archive of Sexual Behavior* 36: 724–40.

Bieber, I., H.J. Dain, P.R. Dince, M.G. Drellich, H.G. Grand, R.H. Gundlach, M.W. Kremer, A.H. Rifkin, C.B. Wilbur, and T.B. Bieber. 1962. *Homosexuality: A psychoanalytic study.* New York: Basic Books.

Blanchard, R. 2004. "Quantitative and theoretical analyses of the relationship between older brothers and homosexuality in men." *Journal of Theoretical Biology* 230: 173–87.

Blanchard, R., H.E. Barbaree, A.F. Bogarert, R. Dickey, P. Klassen, M.E. Kuban, and K.J. Zucker. 2000. "Fraternal birth order and sexual orientation in pedophiles." *Archives of Sexual Behavior* 5: 463–76.

Blanchard, R., and A.F. Boagaert. 1996. "Homosexuality in men and number of older brothers." *American Journal of Psychiatry* 153: 27–32.

Blanchard, R., M.S. Watson, A. Choy, and R. Dickey. 1999. "Pedophiles: Mental retardation, maternal age, and sexual orientation." *Archives of Sexual Behavior* 28: 111–28.

Blanchard, R., K.J. Zucker, P.T. Cohen-Kettenis, L.J.G. Gooren, and J.M. Bailey. 1996. "Birth order and sibling sex ratio in two-samples of Dutch gender-dysphoric homosexual males." *Archives of Sexual Behavior* 25: 495–514.

Bledsoe, L., K. Jay, and S.F. Rogers. 2001. "Sports and lesbian culture." *Gay & Lesbian Review Worldwide* 8(4): 9–11.

Bocklandt, S., S. Horvath, E. Vilain, and D. H. Hamer. 2006. "Extreme skewing of X chromosome inactivation in mothers of homosexual men." *Human Genetics* 118: 691–94.

Bodhi, B., ed. 2005. *In the Buddha's words: An anthology of discourses from the Pali Canon.* Boston: Wisdom.

Boslaugh, S. 2006. "Locating demographic information on GLBT people: A guide to the available reference sources." Paper presented at the GLBT ALMS 2006, International GLBT Archives, Libraries, Museums and Special Collections Conference, May 26, in Minneapolis, MN. http://sfpl.org/librarylocations/main/glc/pdf/glbtdemogboslaugh.pdf.

Boswell, J. 1980. *Christianity, social tolerance, and homosexuality.* Chicago: University of Chicago.

Boswell, J. 1989. "Revolutions, universals, and sexual categories." In *Hidden from history: Reclaiming the gay and lesbian past,* ed. M. B. Duberman, M. Vicinus, and G. Chauncey, pp. 17–36. New York: New American Library.

Boswell, J. 1995. *Same-sex unions in pre-modern Europe.* New York: Villard.

Boyer, P. S., C. E. Clark, S. N. Hawley, J. F. Kett, N. Salisbury, H. Sitkoff, and N. Woloch. 2004. *The enduring vision: A history of the American people.* 5th ed. Boston: Houghton Mifflin.

Bradley, R. H. 2006. As quoted in *MassResistance Watch,* March 23. http://massresistancewatch.blogspot.com/2006/03/letter-from-kris.html.

Bramly, S. 1994. *Leonardo: The artist and the man.* New York: Penguin.

Bray, A. 1996. "To be a man in early modern society: The curious case of Michael Wigglesworth." *History Workshop Journal* 41: 155–65.

Brooks, D. 2004. "The power of marriage." In *Same sex marriage: Pro and con,* ed. Andrew Sullivan, pp. 196–98. New York: Vintage.

Brubaker, L. L. 2002. "Comment on Cameron and Cameron: Children of homosexual parents report childhood difficulties." *Psychological Reports* 91: 331–32.

Bruder, C. E. G., A. Piotrowski, A. Gijsbers, R. Andersson, et al. 2008. "Phenotypically concordant and discordant monozygotic *twins* display different DNA copy-number-variation profiles." *American Journal of Human Genetics* 82: 763–71.

Byne, W. 1995. "Science and belief: Psychobiological research on sexual orientation." *Journal of Homosexuality* 28: 303–44.

Byne, W., S. Tobet, L. A. Mattiace, M. S. Lasco, E. Kemether, M. A. Edgar, S. Morgello, M. S. Buchsbaum, and L. B. Jones. 2001. "The interstitial nuclei of the human anterior hypothalamus: An investigation of variation with sex, sexual orientation, and HIV status." *Hormones and Behavior* 40: 86–92.

Cameron, P. 2006. "Children of homosexuals and transsexuals more apt to be homosexual." *Journal of Biosocial Sciences* 38: 413–18.

Carlson, H. 2003. "A methodological critique of Spitzer's research on reparative therapy." *Archives of Sexual Behavior* 32: 423–27.

Carlson, M. 1998. "Praying away the gay." *Time Magazine* 152(4): 16.

Caramagno, T.C. 2002. *Irreconcilable differences? Intellectual stalemate in the gay rights debate.* Westport, CT: Praeger.

Cassidy, L. 2006. "That many of us should not parent." *Hypathia* 21(4): 40–58.

Cianciotto, J., and S. Cahill. 2006. *Youth in crosshairs: The third wave of ex-gay activism.* Washington, D.C.: National Gay and Lesbian Task Force Policy Institute.

Clark, S.J. 2006. "Gay priests and other boogey men." *Journal of Homosexuality* 51(4): 1–13.

Cloud, J. 2008. "Prosecuting the gay teen murder." *Time Online.* http://www.time.com/time/nation/article/0,8599,1714214,00.html.

Cloud, J. October 2, 2005. "The battle over gay teens." *Time Magazine.* http://www.time.com/time/magazine/article/0,9171,1112856-2,00.html.

Cohen, K.M. 2003. "Are converts to be believed? Assessing sexual orientation 'conversion.'" *Archives of Sexual Behavior* 32: 427–29.

Cole, S.S., and T.M. Cole. 1999. "Sexual, disability, and reproduction issues through the lifespan." In *The psychological and social impact of disability,* ed. R.P. Marinelli and A.E. Dell Orto, pp. 241–56. New York: Springer.

Cones, B. 2006. "Vatican family council goes on the offensive." *U.S. Catholic* 71 (August): 8–9.

Conrad, P., and A. Angell. 2004. "Homosexuality and remedicalization." *Society* 41(5): 32–39.

Council for Responsible Genetics. 2006. "Brief on sexual orientation and genetic determinism." http://www.councilforresponsiblegenetics.org/ViewPage.aspx?pageId=66 .

Courage. 2000a. "The Courage apostolate." http://couragerc.net/TheCourageApostolate.html.

Courage. 2000b. "The five goals." http://couragerc.net/ TheFiveGoals.html.

Crompton, L. 2003. *Homosexuality & civilization.* Cambridge, MA: Belknap Press.

Curry, G.E. 2007. "Jerry Falwell's racist past." *Frost Illustrated,* May 5. http://www.frostillustrated.com/printfull.php?sid=1384.

Cuskelly, M., and R. Bryde. 2004. "Attitudes towards the sexuality of adults with an intellectual disability: Parents, support staff, and a community sample." *Journal of Intellectual and Developmental Disability* 29: 255–64.

De la Huerta, C. 1999. *Coming out spiritually: The next step.* New York: Jeremy Tarcher/Penguin.

Drescher, J. 2003. "The Spitzer study and the culture wars." *Archives of Sexual Behavior* 32: 429–32.

DeSilva, A.L. n.d. "Homosexuality and Theravada Buddhism." *Buddha Net's Magazine.* http://www.buddhanet.net/ homosexu.htm .

Diamond, L. 2003. "What does sexual orientation orient? A biobehavioral model distinguishing romantic love and sexual desire." *Psychological Review* 110: 173–92.

Diamond, L. 2007. "A dynamical systems approach to the development and expression of female same-sex sexuality." *Perspectives on Psychological Science* 2: 142–61.

Dobson, J. 2007. *Marriage under fire: Why we must win this battle.* Carol Stream, IL: Tyndale House Publishers.

Dode, L. 2004. *A history of homosexuality.* Oxford: Trafford Publishing.

Duberman, M. B., M. Vicinus, and G. Chauncey, ed. 1989. *Hidden from history: Reclaiming the gay and lesbian past.* New York: New American Library.

Dunkle, S. W. 1991. "Head damage from mating attempts in dragonflies (odonata; anisoptera)." *Entomological News* 102: 37–41.

Edsall, T. B. 1998. "Forecasting havoc for Orlando; On TV, Robertson says display of gays' flags invites disaster." *The Washington Post,* final edition, June 10, p. A11.

Edwards, J. H., T. Dent, and J. Kahn. 1966. "Monozygotic twins of different sex." *Journal of Medical Genetics* 3: 117–23.

Egan, P. J., M. S. Edelman, and K. Sherrill. 2008. *Findings from the Hunter College poll of lesbians, gays and bisexuals: New discoveries about identities, political attitudes, and civic engagement.* New York: Hunter College.

Ehrlich, P. R. 2002. *Human natures: Genes, cultures, and the human prospect.* New York: Penguin.

El-Rouagher, K. 2005. *Before homosexuality in the Arab Islamic world.* Chicago: University of Chicago.

Elmslie, B., and E. Tebaldi. 2007. "Sexual orientation and labor market discrimination." *Journal of Labor Research* 28: 436–53.

Erens, B., S. McManus, A. Prescott, and J. Field. 2001. *National survey of sexual attitudes and lifestyles II: Reference tables and summary report.* England: National Centre for Social Research.

Erzen, T. 2006. *Straight to Jesus: Sexual and Christian conversions in the ex-gay movement.* Berkeley: University of California Press.

Ettlebrick, P. 2004. "Since when is marriage a path to liberation." In *Same sex marriage: Pro and con,* ed. Andrew Sullivan, pp. 122–28. New York: Vintage.

Evangelical Press.2002. "Ex-gay leader disciplined for gay bar visit." *Christianity Today,* October 1. http://www.christianitytoday.com/ct/2000/octoberweb-only/53.0.html.

Evans, L. October 2002. *Gay chronicles.* http://www.geocities.com/gueroperro/GayChronicles.

Family Equality Council. 2008. "State-by-state: Anti-bullying laws in the U.S." http://www.familyequality.org/resources/publications/anti-bullying_withcitations.pdf.

Florida, R. 2008. *Who's your city: How creative economy is making where to live the most important decision in life,* pp. 136–39. New York: Basic Books.

Floyd, K., J. E. Sargent, and M. DiCorcia. 2004. "Human affection exchange: VI. Further tests of reproductive probability as a predictor of men's affection with their adult sons." *The Journal of Social Psychology* 144: 191–207.

Fone, B. 2000. *Homophobia: A history.* New York: Picador.

Ford, C. S., and F. A. Beach. 1951. *Patterns of sexual behavior.* New York: Harper.

Ford, J. G. 2000. "Reparative therapy is neither." http://www.jgford.homestead. com/fordessay.html.

Fortunata, B., and C. S. Kohn. 2003. "Demographic, psychosocial, and personality characteristics of lesbian batters." *Violence and Victims* 18: 557–69.

French, L. 1992. "Characteristics of sexuality within correctional environments." *Corrective and Social Psychiatry and Journal of Behavior Technology Methods and Therapy* 38: 5–8.

Friedman, R. C. 2003. "Sexual orientation change: A study of atypical cases." *Archives of Sexual Behavior* 32: 432–33.

Friedman, R. C., and J. I. Downey. 2007. "Sexual orientation: Neuroendocrine and psychodynamic influences." *Psychiatric Times* 24(2): 47–48.

Frost, D. M., and I. H. Meyer. 2009. "Internalized homophobia and relationship quality among *lesbians,* gay men, and bisexuals." *Journal of Counseling Psychology* 56: 97–109.

Furth, B., and G. Hoffman. 2006. "Social grease for female? Same-sex genital contacts in wild bonobos." In *Homosexual behaviour in animals: An evolutionary perspective,* ed. V. Sommer and P. L. Vasey, pp. 294–316. Cambridge: Cambridge University.

Gallup, G. G. 1995. "Have attitudes toward homosexuals been shaped by natural selection?" *Ethology and Sociobiology* 16: 53–70.

Garber, E. 1989. "A spectacle in color: The lesbian and gay subculture of jazz age Harlem." In *Hidden from history: Reclaiming the gay and lesbian past,* ed. M. B. Duberman, M. Vicinus, and G. Chauncey, pp. 90–105. New York: New American Library.

Garber, L. 2003. "Lesbian feminism." In *Lesbian histories and cultures: An encyclopedia,* ed. B. Zimmerman, pp. 456–59. New York: Garland.

Gardner, F. 2006. "Nixon on pot, booze and the fall of the Roman Empire." *CounterPunch,* December 30. http://www.counterpunch.org/gardner12302006. html.

Garner, A. 2004. *Families like mine: Children of gay parents tell it like it is.* New York: Harper Collins.

Garofalo, R., C. Wolf, L. S. Wissow, E. R. Woods, and E. Goodman. 1999. "Sexual orientation and risk of suicide attempts among a representative sample of youth." *Archives of Pediatric Adolescent Medicine* 153: 487–93. http://arch pedi.ama-assn.org/cgi/content/abstract/153/5/487.

Gill, G. 2004a. *Nightingales: The extraordinary upbringing and curious life of Miss Florence Nightingale.* New York: Ballantine.

Gill, G. 2004b. Appearing on *The Diane Rehm Show,* October 14. http://home. wamu.org/programs/dr/04/10/14.php?displayStatus=show.

GLAAD. n.d. "Media reference guide." http://www.glaad.org/referenceguide.

Gliding, H. M. D., P. F. Bolton, J. Vincent, G. Melmer, and M. Rutter. 1997. "Molecular and cytogenetic investigations of the fragile X region including the

Frax A and Frax E CGG trinucleotide repeat sequences in families multiplex for autism and related phenotypes." *Human Heredity* 47: 254–62.

Goldberg, J. 2005. "Aborting ideology as we know it." *National Review Online,* February 25. http://www.nationalreview.com/goldberg/goldberg2005022 50924.asp.

Goldstein, M.A. 2003. "Male puberty: Physical, psychological, and emotional issues." *Adolescent Medicine* 14: 541–54.

Gottlieb, A.R. 2003. *Sons talk about their gay fathers: Life curves.* Binghamton, NY: Harrington Park Press.

Green, R. 1988. "The immutability of (homo)sexual orientation: Behavioral science implications for constitutional (legal) analysis." *Journal of Psychiatry* 16: 537–76.

Greenberg, D.F. 1988. *The construction of homosexuality.* Chicago: University of Chicago Press.

Griffin, P., and M. Ouellett. 2003. "From silence to safety and beyond: Historical trends in addressing lesbian, gay, bisexual, transgender issues in K–12 schools." *Equality & Excellence in Education* 36: 106–14.

Groth, A.N., and A.W. Burgess. 1980. "Male rape: Offenders and victims." *American Journal of Psychiatry* 137: 806–810.

Gunderson, S., and R. Morris. 1996. *House and home.* New York: E. P. Dutton.

Haddock, G., and M.P. Zanna. 1998. "Authoritarianism, values, and the favorability and structure of antigay attitudes." In *Stigma and sexual orientation: Understanding prejudice against, lesbians, gay men, and bisexuals,* ed. G. M. Herek, pp. 82–107. Thousand Oaks, CA: Sage.

Haeberle, E.J. 1989. "Swastika, pink triangle and yellow star: The destruction of sexology and the persecution of homosexuals in Nazi Germany." In *Hidden from history: Reclaiming the gay and lesbian past,* ed. M.B. Duberman, M. Vicinus, and G. Chauncey, pp. 365–79. New York: New American Library.

Haldeman, D. C. 1994. "The practice and ethics of sexual orientation conversion therapy." *Journal of Consulting and Clinical Psychology* 62: 221–27.

Haldeman, D. C. 1999. "The pseudo-science of sexual-orientation conversion therapy." *Angles: The Policy Journal of the Institute for Gay and Lesbian Strategic Studies* 4: 1–4.

Haldeman, D. C. 2004. "When sexual and religious orientation collide: Considerations in working with conflicted same-sex attracted male clients." *The Counseling Psychologist* 32: 691–715.

Hall, J., and D. Kimura. 1995. Sexual orientation and performance on sexually dimorphic motor tasks. *Archives of Sexual Behavior* 24: 395–407.

Hall, J.A.Y., and D. Kimura. 1994. "Dermatoglyphic asymmetry and sexual orientation in men." *Behavioral Neuroscience* 108: 1203–6.

Hall, L. S., and C.T. Love. 2003. "Finger-length ratios in female monozygotic twins discordant for sexual orientation." *Archives of Sexual Behavior* 32: 23–29.

Hall, P.A., and C.M. Schaeff. 2008. "Sexual orientation and fluctuating asymmetry in men and women." *Archives of Sexual Behavior* 37: 158–65.

Hall, R.C.W., and R.C.W. Hall. 2007. "A profile of pedophilia: Definition, characteristics of offenders, recidivism, treatment outcomes, and forensic issues." *Mayo Clinic Proceedings* 82: 457–72.

Hallman, J.M. 2005. "Helping women with same-sex attraction." *NARTH Bulletin* 13(1): 33–36.

Halperin, D. 1989. "Sex before sexuality: Pederasty, politics and power in classical Athens." In *Hidden from history: Reclaiming the gay and lesbian past,* ed. M.B. Duberman, M. Vicinus, and G. Chauncey, pp. 37–53. New York: New American Library.

Hamer, D., and P. Copeland. 1998. *Living with our genes.* New York: Anchor.

Hamer, D.H., S. Hu, V.L. Magnuson, N. Hu, and A.M.L. Pattatucci. 1993. "A linkage between DNA markers on the X chromosome and male sexual orientation." *Science* 21: 321–27.

Hari, J. 2008. "The strange, strange story of the gay fascists." *Huffington Post,* October 21. http://www.huffingtonpost.com/johann-hari/the-strange-strange-story_b_136697.html.

Harris, S. 2005. *The end of faith: Religion, terror, and the future of reason.* New York: W.W. Norton.

Harris Interactive Inc. 2005. *From teasing to torment: School climate in America.* New York: GLSEN.

Harris Interactive Inc. 2008. *The principal's perspective: School safety, bullying and harassment a survey of public school principals.* New York: GLSEN.

Hartmann, L. 2003. "Too flawed, don't publish." *Archives of Sexual Behavior* 32: 346–47.

Harvey, P. 2000. *Introduction to Buddhist ethics.* Cambridge, UK: Cambridge University.

Harvey, J.F. 1996. *The truth about homosexuality: Comprehensive view of the issues involved in homosexuality.* San Francisco: Ignatius.

Hawkins, D.N., and A. Booth. 2005. "Unhappily ever after: Effects of long-term, low-quality marriages on well-being." *Social Forces* 84(1): 451–72.

Hecht, P. 2008. "Field Poll: Majority of Californians now support gay marriage." *The Sacramento Bee,* May 28. http://www.sacbee.com/111/story/970055.html.

Heller, D. 2003. "Feminism." In *Lesbian histories and cultures: An encyclopedia,* ed. B. Zimmerman, pp. 293–94. New York: Garland.

Hendrickson, M. 2005. "Lavender parents." *Social Policy Journal of New Zealand* 26: 68–84.

Henry, G.W. *Sex Variants: A Study of Homosexual Patterns.* New York: Hoeber.

Herdt, G.H., and R.J. Stoller. 1989. "Commentary to socialization of homosexuality in a non-western society." *Archives of Sexual Behavior* 18: 31–34.

Heredity. 2008. *Encyclopedia Britannica.* http://www.britannica.com/EBchecked/topic/262934/heredity.

Herek, G.M. 2003a. "Evaluating interventions to alter sexual orientation: Method-ological and ethical considerations." *Archives of Sexual Behavior* 32: 337–39.

Herek, G. M. 2003b. "The psychology of sexual prejudice." In *Psychological per-spectives on lesbian, gay, and bisexual experiences,* ed. L.M. Garnets and D. C. Kimmel, pp. 157–64. New York: Columbia University.

Herek, G. M. n.d. "Paul Cameron bio and fact sheet." http://psychology.ucdavis.edu/rainbow/html/facts_cameron_sheet.html#note5_text.

Herman, D. 1997. *The antigay agenda: Orthodox vision and the Christian right.* Chicago: University of Chicago Press.

Hinsch, B. 1990. *Passion of the cut sleeve: The male homosexual tradition in China.* Berkeley: University of California.

Hodel, D. 1993. "A lesson of happiness: Anyone can achieve it says the Dali Lama to Seattle crowd." *World Tibet Network News,* July 31. http://community.seattletimes.nwsource.com/archive/?date=19930629&slug=1708730.

Holland, E. 2004. *The nature of homosexuality: Vindication for the homosexual ac-tivist and the religious right,* pp. 352–71. New York: Universe.

Howey, N., and E. Samuels. 2000. *Out of the ordinary: Essays on growing up with gay, lesbian, and transgender parents.* New York: St. Martin's.

Hu, S., A. Pattatucci, C. Patterson, L. Li, D. Fulker, S. Cherny, L. Kruglyak, and D. Hamer. 1995. "Linkage between sexual orientation and chromosome Xq28 in males, but not females." *Natural Genetics* 11: 248–56.

Hubbard, T.K., ed. 2003. Introduction in *Homosexuality in Greece and Rome: A sourcebook of basic documents,* pp. 1–20. Berkeley: University of Cali-fornia.

Hull, K. 2005. "Employment discrimination based on sexual orientation: dimen-sions of difference." In *Handbook of employment discrimination research: Rights and realities.*], ed. L.B. Nielsen and R.L. Nelson, pp. 167–87. New York: Springer.

Human Rights Campaign. 2007. "GLBT equality at the Fortune 500." http://www.hrc.org/issues/workplace/fortune500.htm.

Human Rights Campaign. 2009a. "GLBT equality at the Fortune 500." http://www.hrc.org/issues/workplace/fortune500.htm.

Human Rights Campaign. 2009b. "Timeline: The Employment Non-Discrimination Act." http://www.hrc.org/issues/workplace/5636.htm.

Human Rights Campaign. 2009c. "Workplace: Laws." http://www.hrc.org/issues/workplace/workplace_laws.asp.

Human Rights Watch. 2005. "Iran: Two more executions for homosexual conduct." *Human Rights News,* November 22. http://www.hrw.org/en/news/2005/11/21/iran-two-more-executions-homosexual-conduct.

International Lesbian and Gay Association. 2000. "World legal survey." http://ilga.org/ilga/en/Articles?select=tag:world legal survey.

Jaschik, S. 2008. "Michigan ruling bars domestic partner benefits." *Inside Higher Ed,* May 8. http://www.insidehighered.com/news/2008/05/08/benefits.

Jenny, C., T.A. Roesler, and K.L. Poyer. 1994. "Are children at risk of sexual abuse by homosexuals?" *Pediatrics* 94: 41–44.

Johnson, A. M., J. Wadsworth, K. Wellings, and J. Field. 1994. *Sexual attitudes and lifestyles.* Oxford: Blackwell Scientific Publications.

JOHAH. 2001. "JONAH: Jews offering new alternatives to homosexuality." http://www.jonahweb.org/index.php.

Josephus, F. 1988. "Jewish Antiquities." *Josephus: The essential writings.* Trans. and ed. P.L. Maier. Original work published circa 93 c.e. Grand Rapids, MI: Kregel.

Katz, J. 1976. *Gay American history.* New York: Thomas Y. Crowell.

Kemkes-Grottenthaler, A. 2003. "Postponing or rejecting parenthood? Results of a survey among female academic professionals." *Journal of Biosocial Science* 35: 213–26.

Kendler, K. S., L. M. Thornton, S. E. Gilman, and R. C. Kessler. 2000. "Sexual orientation in a national sample of twin and nontwin pairs." *The American Journal of Psychiatry* 157: 1843–47.

Kennedy, J. 2003. "John Geddes Lawrence and Tyron Garner, petitioners v. Texas." http://caselaw.lp.findlaw.com/scripts/getcase.pl?court=US&vol=000&invol=02-102#dissent1.

King, J. L., and K. Hunter. 2004. *On the down low: A journey into the lives of "straight" black men who sleep with men.* New York: Broadway Books, 2004.

King, M. L. 1964. *Why we can't wait.* New York: Harper & Row.

Kinsey, A. C., W. B. Pomeroy, and C. Martin C. 1948. *Sexual behavior in the human male.* Philadelphia: W. B. Saunders.

Kirk, K. M., J. M. Bailey, M. P. Dunne, and N. G. Martin. 2000. "Measurement models for sexual orientation in a community twin sample." *Behavior Genetics* 30: 345–56.

Kirk, M., and H. Madsen. 1989. *After the ball: How America will conquer its fear and hatred of gays in the '90s.* New York: Doubleday.

Kirk, R. C. 2000. "The evolution of human homosexual behavior." *Current Anthropology* 41: 385–417.

Kite, M. E., and B. E. Whitley. 1998. "Do women and men differ in their attitudes toward homosexuality? A conceptual and methodological analysis." In *Stigma and sexual orientation: Understanding prejudice against, lesbians, gay men, and bisexuals,* ed. G. M. Herek, pp. 39–61. Thousand Oaks, CA: Sage.

Kligerman, N. 2007. "Homosexuality in Islam: A difficult paradox." *Macalester Islam Journal* 2(3): 52–64. http://www.asylumlaw.org/docs/sexualminorities/HomosexualityinIslam0407.pdf.

Kosciw, J. G., E. M. Diaz, and E. A. Greytak. 2008. "The experiences of lesbian, gay, bisexual and transgender youth in our nation's schools." *The 2007 national school climate survey: The experiences of lesbian, gay, bisexual and transgender youth in our nation's schools.* New York: GLSEN.

Kotrschal, K., J. Hemetsberger, and B. M. Weib. 2006. "Making the best of a bad situation: Homosociology in male greylag geese." In *Homosexual behaviour in animals: An evolutionary perspective,* ed. V. Sommer and P. L. Vasey, pp. 45–76. Cambridge: Cambridge University.

Kovacs, J. 2002. "Kodak fires man over 'gay' stance: 23-year veteran of global film giant objected to pro-homosexual memo." *WorldNetDaily.Com,* October 24. http://www.wnd.com/news/article.asp?ARTICLE_ID=29394.

Kramer, E. J. 1998. "When men are victims: Applying rape shield laws to male same-sex rape." *New York University Law Review* 73: 293–331.

Krstovic, J. 1997. "Sappho: Overview." In *Gay & lesbian biography,* ed. in M. J. Tyrkus. Detroit: St. James Press. http://galenet.galegroup.com.dax.lib.unf.edu/servlet/LitRC?vrsn=3&oldim=1&locID=jack91990&ste=135&docNum=H1420007072.

Kurdek, L. A. 2004. "Are gay and lesbian cohabitating couples really different from heterosexual married couples?" *Journal of Marriage and Family* 66: 880–901.

Lambda Legal. 2009a. *Nabozny v. Podlesny.* http://www.lambdalegal.org/our-work/in-court/cases/nabozny-v-podlesny.html.

Lambda Legal. 2009b. *Noble Street Gay Straight Alliance v. Noble Network of Charter School.* http://www.lambdalegal.org/our-work/in-court/cases/noble-street-gsa-v-noble.html.

Larsson, I. B., and C. G. Svedin. 2002. "Sexual experience in childhood: Young adults' recollections." *Archives of Sexual Behavior* 31: 263–73.

Latham, H. F. 2005. "Desperately clinging to the Cleavers: What family law courts are doing about homosexual parents, and what some are refusing to see." *Law and Psychology Review* 29: 223–42.

Laumann, E. O., J. H. Gagnon, R. T. Michael, and S. Michaels. 1994. *The social organization of sexuality: Sexual practices in the United States.* Chicago: University of Chicago.

Leland, J., and M. Miller. 1998. "Can gays convert?" *Newsweek* 132(7): 46–51.

Leupp, G. P. 1995. *Male colors: The construction of homosexuality in Tokugawa Japan.* Berkeley: University of California.

LeVay, S. 1996. *Queer science.* Cambridge: MIT.

Levina, M., C. R. Waldo, and L. F. Fitzgerald. 2000. *Journal of Applied Social Psychology* 30: 738–58.

Library of Congress. n.d. "Thomas: House Report 110–113—Local Law Enforcement Hate Crimes Prevention Act of 2007." http://www.govtrack.us/congress/bill.xpd?bill=h110-1592

Lipkin, A. 2003. *Beyond diversity day: A Q&A on gay and lesbian issues in schools.* New York: Rowan and Littlefield.

Lively, S. July 2002. "Homosexuality and the Nazi party." *Leadership U.* http://wthrockmorton.com/2009/06/25/leadership-university-removes-homosexuality-and-the-nazi-party-article/.

Locke, K.A. 2004. "The Bible on homosexuality: Exploring its meaning and authority." *Journal of Homosexuality* 48: 125–56.

Loftin, C.M. 2007. "Unacceptable mannerisms: Gender anxieties, homosexual activism, and swish in the United States." *Journal of Social History* 40: 577–96.

"Love with an improper stranger." 1984. *Time Magazine.* http://www.time.com/time/magazine/article/0,9171,953455-1,00.html.

Lynch, P.E. 2006. "An interview with Ralph E. Roughton, M.D." *Journal of Gay and Lesbian Psychotherapy* 10(2): 105–16.

Malebranche, J. 2006. *Androphilia: A manifesto.* Baltimore: Scapegoat.

Mann, J. 2006. "Establishing trust: Socio-sexual behaviour and the development of male-male bonds among Indian Ocean bottlenose dolphins." In *Homosexual behaviour in animals: An evolutionary perspective,* ed. V. Sommer and P.L. Vasey, pp. 107–30. Cambridge: Cambridge University Press.

Martins, Y., G. Preti, C.R. Crabtree, T. Runyan, A.A. Vainius, and C.J. Wysocki. 2005. "Preference for human body odors is influenced by gender and sexual orientation." *Psychological Science* 16: 694–701.

Massachusetts Department of Education. 1995. "Gay/straight alliances: A student guide recommendations on the support and safety of gay and lesbian students." http://www.doe.mass.edu/cnp/GSA/safegl.html.

Massachusetts Department of Education. 2001. "Education laws and regulations." http://www.doe.mass.edu/lawsregs/603cmr26.html?section=all.

Massachusetts Department of Education. 2007. "The safe schools program for gay & lesbian students." http://www.doe.mass.edu/cnp/safe/ssch.html.

Massey, M. 1988. *Women in ancient Greece and Rome.* Cambridge: Cambridge University.

McClennen, J.C. 2005. "Domestic violence between same-gender partners: Research findings and future research." *Journal of Interpersonal Violence* 20: 149–54.

McLaren, B.D. 2006. *The secret message of Jesus: Uncovering the truth that could change everything.* Nashville, TN: Thomas Nelson.

McNeill, J.J. 1993. *The church and the homosexual.* Boston: Beacon Hill.

Meacham, J. 2006. *American gospel: God, the founding fathers, and making of a nation.* New York: Random House.

Medinger, A. 2000. *Growth into manhood: Resuming the journey.* Colorado Springs: Water Brook Press.

Meijer, M.M., F.P.M. Ewals, and F.A. Scholte. 2003. "Health Council of the Netherlands' report on contraception in intellectually disabled people." *Nederlands tijdschrift voor geneeskunde* 147(5): 188–91.

Mencimer, S. June 2001. "The baby boycott." *The Washington Monthly* 33(6): 14–19.

Mercurio, M.A., and C.R.A. Morse. 2007. "Tinkering close to the edge." *Educational Leadership* 64: 52–5.

Moberly, E.R. 1983. *Homosexuality: A new Christian ethic.* Cambridge, England: James Clark.

Mohler, A. 2007. "Is your baby gay? What if you could know? What if you could do something about it?" *The Albert Mohler Radio Program,* March 2. http://www.albertmohler.com/radio_show.php?cdate=2007-03-07.

Morrow, S.L., and A.L. Beckstead. 2004. "Conversion therapies for same-sex attracted clients in religious conflict: Context, predisposing, factors, experiences, and implications for therapy." *The Counseling Psychologist* 32: 641–50.

Morrison, T.G. 2007. "Debate—Children of homosexuals and transsexuals more apt to be homosexual: A reply to Cameron." *Journal of Biosocial Sciences* 39: 153–54.

Mullen, K. 1996. "Marital status and men's health." *The International Journal of Sociology and Social Policy* 16(3): 47–68.

Murray, J.B. 2000 "Psychological profile of pedophiles and child molesters." *The Journal of Psychology* 134: 211–25.

Murray, S. 2000. *Homosexualities.* Chicago: University of Chicago.

Musbach, T. 2005. "Roy and Silo famous pair no more." *The Advocate: News and Politics,* September 8.

Muscarella, F. 2002. "Homoerotic behavior in human evolution." *The Gay & Lesbian Review* 9(6): 14–18.

Mustanski, B.S., M.L. Chivers, and J.M. Bailey. 2002. "A critical review of recent biological research on human sexual orientation." *Annual Review of Sex Research* 13: 89–140.

Mustanski, B.S., M.G. Dupree, C.M. Nievergelt, S. Bocklandt, N.J. Schork, and D. Hamer. 2005. "A genomewide scan of male sexual orientation." *Human Genetics* 116: 272–78.

Myers, D.G., and L.D. Scanzoni. 2005. *What God has joined together? A Christian case for gay marriage.* San Francisco: Harper.

National Association of Research and Therapy of Homosexuality. 2004. "The A.P.A. Normalization of Homosexuality, and the Research Study of Irving Bieber." http://www.narth.com/docs/normalization.html.

National Education Association. 1975. *Code of ethics.* http://www.nea.org/home/30442.htm.

National Gay and Lesbian Task Force. n.d. "Archaic Sex Laws." http://www.thetaskforce.org/issues/nondiscrimination/sodomy.

Negy, C., and R. Eisenman. 2005. "A comparison of African American and white college students' affective and attitudinal reactions to lesbians, gay, and bisexual individuals: An exploratory study." *The Journal of Sex Research* 43: 291–98.

Nelson, N. 2004. "The majority of cancers are linked to the environment." *Benchmark* 4 (June 17): 3. http://www.cancer.gov/templates/doc_bench.aspx?viewid=5d17e03e-b39f-4b40-a214-e9e9099c4220&docid=4ed11bf0-c7eb-4797-95f3-049be19a8fa2&print=1.

New Hope Ministries. n.d. "Steps Out Residential Program: September 6–November 20, 2007." http://www.newhope123.org/residential.htm.

Ng, V.W. 1989. "Homosexuality and the state in late imperial China." In *Hidden from history: Reclaiming the gay and lesbian past,* ed. M.B. Duberman, M. Vicinus, and G. Chauncey, pp. 76–89. New York: New American Library.

Nicolosi, J. 2009. "The meaning of same-sex attraction."http://www.narth.com/docs/niconew.html.

Nicolosi, J. 2002. "Efforts to silence NARTH continue." *Leadership U,* July 14. http://www.leaderu.com/orgs/narth/efforts.html.

Newton, E. 1989. "The mythic mannish, lesbian: Radclyffe Hall and the new women." In *Hidden from history: Reclaiming the gay and lesbian past,* ed. M.B. Duberman, M. Vicinus, and G. Chauncey, pp. 281–93. New York: New American Library.

North American Man/Boy Love Association. 2003. "Who are we." http://nambla.org/welcome.htm.

Ohms, C. 2008. "Perpetrators of violence and abuse in lesbian partnerships." *Liverpool Law Review* 29: 81–97.

Panate, V. 2006. "Homosexuality in the Middle East and North Africa." *Gay life and culture: A world history,* ed. R. Aldrich, pp. 270–301. London: Thames & Hudson.

Parker, I. 2007. "Swingers." *The New Yorker,* July 30. http://www.newyorker.com/reporting/2007/07/30/070730fa_fact_parker?currentPage=all.

Parnell, P., and Justin Richardson. 2005. *And Tango makes three.* New York: Simon and Schuster.

Partners Task Force for Gay and Lesbian Couples.2007. "Domestic partnership benefits: Philosophy and providers list." http://www.buddybuddy.com/d-p-1.html.

Pattison, E.M., and M.L. Pattison. 1980. "Ex-gays: Religiously mediated change in homosexuals." *American Journal of Psychiatry* 137: 1153–62.

Pew Research Center. 2007. "The Pew global attitudes project: Spring 2007 survey." http://pewglobal.org/reports/pdf/258topline.pdf.

Phelps, D. n.d. "Flexing muscle: How the 2004 gay vote will make a difference." *GayToday.* http://www.gaytoday.com/penpoints/062804pp.asp.

Pinckard, K.J., J. Stellflug, J.A. Resko, C.E. Roselli, and F. Stormshak. 2000. "Review: Brain armomatization and other factors affecting male reproductive behavior with emphasis on the sexual orientation of rams." *Domestic Animal Endocrinology* 18: 83–96.

Plöderl, M., and R. Fartacek. 2009. "Childhood gender nonconformity and harassment as predictors of suicidality among gay, lesbian, bisexual, and heterosexual Austrians." *Archives of Sexual Behavior* 38: 400–410.

Popenoe, D. 2007. "Top 10 marriage myths. Love & Relationships." *Discovery Health.* http://health.discovery.com/centers/loverelationships/articles/marriage_myths.html.

Powledge, T. M. 1993. "The inheritance of behavior in twins." *Bioscience* 43: 420–25.

Purcell, D. W., R. Blanchard, and K. J. Zucker. 2000. "Birth order in a contemporary sample of gay men." *Archives of Sexual Behavior* 29: 349–56.

Quinnipiac University Polling Institute. 2008. "American voters oppose same-sex marriage Quinnipiac University national poll finds, but they don't want government to ban it." http://www.quinnipiac.edu/x1295.xml?ReleaseID=1194.

Radow, R. 1994. "NAMBLA Replies to ILGA Secretariat (Revised)." http://www.qrd.org/qrd/orgs/NAMBLA/nambla.replies.to.ilga.secretariat.

Rahman, Q., G. D. Wilson, and S. Abrahams. 2003. "Sexual orientation related differences in spatial memory." *Journal of International Neuropsychological Society* 9: 376–83.

Ratzinger, J. 1986. "A letter to the bishops of the Catholic Church on the pastoral care of homosexual persons." http://www.vatican.va/roman_curia/congregations/cfaith/documents/rc_con_cfaith_doc_19861001_homosexual-persons_en.html.

Reeder, G. 2000. "Same-sex desire, conjugal constructs, and the tomb of Niankhkhnum and Khnumhotep." *World Archaeology* 32: 193–208.

Remafedi, G., S. French, M. Story, M. D. Resnick, and R. Blum. 1998. "The relationship between suicide risk and sexual orientation: Results of a population-based study." *American Journal of Public Health* 88: 57–60. http://www.ajph.org/cgi/content/abstract/88/1/57.

Rice, G., C. Anderson, N. Risch, and G. Ebers. 1999. "Male homosexuality: Absence of linkage to microsatellite markers at Xq28." *Science* 284: 665–68.

Robertson, P. 2007. "700 Club: So-called 'gay-agenda' on West Coast." *The 700 Club,* December 14. http://www.youtube.com/watch?v=VvPGZ56LBd8.

Robitaille, C., and M. Saint-Jacques. 2009. "Social stigma and situation of young people in lesbian and gay stepfamilies." *Journal of Homosexuality* 56: 421–42.

Rondeau, P. E. 2002. "Selling homosexuality to America." *Regent University Law Review* 14: 443–85.

Roselli, C. E., K. Larkin, J. M. Schrunk, and F. Stormshak. 2004. "Sexual partner preference, hypothalamic morphology and aromatase in rams." *Physiology & Behavior* 83: 233–45.

Roselli, C. E., J. A. Resko, and F. Stormshak. 2002. "Hormonal influences on sexual partner preference in rams." *Archives of Sexual Behavior* 31: 43–49.

Rowe, R. N. 2006. "Homosexual teachers in the classroom: The debate continues." *Clearing House: A Journal of Educational Strategies, Issues and Ideas* 79(5): 207–8.

Russell, S. T., and K. Joyner. 2001. "Adolescent sexual orientation and suicide risk: Evidence from a national study." *American Journal of Public Health* 91: 1276–81. http://www.pubmedcentral.nih.gov/articlerender.fcgi?artid=1446760.

Rutter, P. A., and E. Soucar. 2002. "Youth suicide risk and sexual orientation—Statistical data included." *Adolescence,* Summer. http://findarticles.com/p/articles/mi_m2248/is_146_37/ai_89942832.

Ryan C., D. Huebner, R. M. Diaz, and J. Sanchez. 2009. "Family rejection as a predictor of negative health outcomes in white and Latino lesbian, gay, and bisexual young adults." *Pediatrics* 123: 346–52.

Saad, L. 2008. "Americans evenly divided on morality of homosexuality: However majority supports legality and acceptance of gay relationships." Princeton: Gallup. http://www.gallup.com/poll/108115/Americans-Evenly-Divided-Morality-Homosexuality.aspx.

Sageman, S. 2003. "The rape of boys and the impact of sexually predatory environments: Review and case reports." *Journal of the American Academy of Psychoanalysis and Dynamic Psychiatry* 31: 563–80.

Salzman, T. A., and M. E. Lawler. 2006. "Catholic sexual ethics: Complementarity and truly human." *Theological Studies* 67: 625–52.

Santosuosso, A. 2004. *Barbarians, marauders and infidels: The ways of medieval warfare.* Boulder: Westview Press.

Saslow, J. W. 1989. "Homosexuality in the renaissance: Behavior, identity and artistic expression." In *Hidden from history: Reclaiming the gay and lesbian past,* ed. M. B. Duberman, M. Vicinus, and G. Chauncey, pp. 90–105. New York: New American Library.

Satcher, J., and M. Leggett, M. 2007. "Homonegativity among professional school counselors: An exploratory study." *Professional School Counseling Journal* 11: 10–16.Savage, M. 2006. *The savage nation.* Mill Valley, CA: The Paul Revere Society, as heard on the Talk Radio Network.

Savic, I., H. Berglund, and P. Lindström. 2005. "Brain response to putative pheromones in homosexual men." *Proceedings of the National Academy of Sciences of the United States of America* 102: 7356–61.

Savin-Williams, R. C. 2005. *The new gay teenager.* Cambridge, MA: Harvard University.

Scalia, A. 2003. *John Geddes Lawrence and Tyron Garner, Petitioners v. Texas.* http://caselaw.lp.findlaw.com/scripts/getcase.pl?court=US&vol=000&invol=02-102#dissent1.

Schalow, P. G. 1989. "Male love in early modern Japan: A literary depiction of the 'Youth.'" In *Hidden from history: Reclaiming the gay and lesbian past,* ed. M. B. Duberman, M. Vicinus, and G. Chauncey, pp. 118–28. New York: New American Library.

Schmitt, D. P. 2006. "Sexual strategies across sexual orientations: How personality traits and culture relate to sociosexuality among gays, lesbians, bisexuals, and heterosexuals." *Journal of Psychology & Human Sexuality* 18: 183–205.

Schwartz, A. E. 1998. *Sexual subjects: Lesbians, gender and psychoanalysis.* New York: Routledge.

Seel, P. 1995. *I, Pierre Seel: deported homosexual.* Trans. Joachim Neugroschel, pp. 42–44. New York: Basic Books.

Sell, R.L., J.A. Wells, and D. Wypij. 1995. "The prevalence of homosexual behavior and attraction in the United State, the United Kingdom, and France: Results of national population-base samples." *Archives of Sexual Behavior* 24: 235–49.

Serwatka, T.S., and L. Carroll. 1999. "Out of the school closet: The invisible minority." In *Ethics in Education,* ed. D. Fenner. New York: Garland Publishing.

Shah, D.K. 2004. "Letter to Senator Bill Frisk, Senate Majority Leader." Washington, D.C.: United States General Accounting Office. http://www.gao.gov/new.items/d04353r.pdf.

Shelton, L.P. 2004. "Constitutional attorney sees polygamy as next stage of sexual revolution." In *Traditional Values Coalition: Inserts,* October 6. www.traditionalvalues.org/inserts/1004Polygamy.pdf .

Shildo, A., and M. Schroder. 2002. "Changing sexual orientation: A consumer's report." *Professional Psychology: Research and Practice* 33: 249–59.

Simon, A. 1998. "The relationship between stereotype and attitudes toward lesbians and gays." In *Stigma and sexual orientation: Understanding prejudice against, lesbians, gay men, and bisexual,* ed. G. M. Herek, pp. 62–81. Thousand Oaks, CA: Sage.

Skidmore, W. C., J.A.W. Linsenmeier, and J.M. Bailey. 2006. "Gender nonconformity and psychological distress in lesbians and gay men." *Archives of Sexual Behavior* 35: 685–97.

Small, M. 1995. *What's love got to do with it: The evolution of human mating.* New York: Anchor.

Smith, D. 2007."Central Park Zoo's gay penguins ignite debate." *New York Times,* February 7, p. A-9.

Smith, A. M.A., C.E. Rissel, J. Richters, A.E. Grulich, and R.O. de Visser. 2003. "Sexual identity, sexual attraction and sexual experience among a representative sample of adults." *Australian and New Zealand Journal of Public Health* 27: 138–45.

Sommer, I.E.C., N.F. Ramsey, R.C.W. Mandl, and R.S. Kahn. 2002. "Language lateralization in monozygotic twin pairs concordant and discordant for handedness." *Brain* 125: 2710–18.

Sommer, V. 2006. "'Against nature?!' An epilogue about animal sex and the moral dimension." In *Homosexual behaviour in animals: An evolutionary perspective,* ed. V. Sommer and P. L. Vasey, pp. 365–71. Cambridge: Cambridge University Press.

Sommer, V., and P.L. Vasey, eds. 2006. *Homosexual behaviour in animals: An evolutionary perspective.* Cambridge: Cambridge University Press.

Spencer, C. 1995. *Homosexuality in history.* New York: Harcourt Brace.

Spitzer, R.L. 2003. "Can some gay men and lesbians change their sexual orientation? 200 participants reporting a change from homosexual to heterosexual orientation." *Archives of Sexual Behavior* 32: 401–17.

Spong, J. S. 2005. *The sins of the scripture: Exposing the Bible's texts of hate to reveal the God of love.* San Francisco: Harper Collins.

Stacey, J., and T. J. Biblarz. 2001. "(How) does the sexual orientation of parents matter." *American Sociological Review* 66: 159–83.

Stack, S., and J. R. Eshleman. 1998. "Marital status and happiness: A 17-nation study." *Journal of Marriage and the Family* 60: 527–37.

Stulhofer, A., and I. Rimac. 2009. "Determinants of homonegativity in Europe." *Journal of Sex Research* 46: 24–32.

Sullivan, A. 1995. *Virtually normal: An argument about homosexuality.* New York: Knopf.

Sullivan, N. 2003. *A critical introduction to queer theory.* New York: New York University Press.

Swift, E. M. 1992. "Dangerous games: In the age of AIDS many pro athletes are sexually promiscuous despite the increasing peril." *Sports Illustrated* 75(22): 40–45.

Swift, M. 1987. "Gay Revolutionary." *Gay Community News,* February 15–21. http://www.fordham.edu/halsall/pwh/swift1.html.

Szymanski, D. M. 2004. "Relations among dimensions of feminism and internalized heterosexism in lesbian and bisexual women." *Sex Roles* 51: 145–59.

Taylor, C. 2009. Interview with Terry Gross. *NPR's Fresh Air.* May 6. http://www.highbeam.com/doc/1P1-166310221.html.

Taywaditep, K. J. 2002. "Marginalization among the marginalized." *Journal of Homosexuality* 4: 1–28.

TFP Committee on American Issues. 2004. *Defending a higher law: Why we must resist same-sex marriage and the homosexual movement.* Spring Grove, PA: American Society for the Defense of Tradition, Family and Property.

Toufexis, A. 1995. "Evidence of a new gay gene." *Time Magazine,* November 13. http://www.time.com/time/magazine/article/0,9171,983713,00.html.

Turner, W. J. 1994. "Comments on discordant monozygotic twinning in homosexuality." *Archives of Sexual Behavior* 23: 115–19.

United States Holocaust Memorial Museum. n.d. *Homosexuals: Victims of Nazi era.* Washington, D.C.

"U.S. Catholics still back birth control." 2006. *Conscience* 27(4): 9. http://find.galegroup.com/itx/infomark.do?&contentSet=IAC-Documents&type=retrieve&tabID=T003&prodId=ITOF&docId=A155404329&source=gale&srcprod=ITOF&userGroupName=jack91990&version=1.0.

U.S. Census Bureau. 2006. "Table H2. Distribution of women over 40 to 45 years old by number of children ever born and marital status: Selected 1970–2004." http://www.census.gov/population/www/socdemo/fertility.html#hist.

U.S. Department of Personnel Management. n.d. *Addressing sexual orientation discrimination in federal civilian employment: A guide to employee's rights.* Washington, D.C. http://www.opm.gov/er/address2/Guide01.asp#Intro.

van der Aardweg. 1986. *On the origins and treatment of homosexuality: A psycho-analytic reinterpretation.* New York: Praeger.

Vasey, P. L. 1995. "Homosexual behavior in primates: A review of evidence and theory." *International Journal of Primatology* 16: 173–204.

Vasey, P. L. 2006. "The pursuit of pleasure: An evolutionary history of homosexual history of homosexual behavior in Japanese macaques." In *Homosexual behaviour in animals: An evolutionary perspective,* ed. V. Sommer and P. L. Vasey, pp. 191–220. Cambridge: Cambridge University Press.

Vasey, P. L. 2006. "Where do you go from here? Research on the evolution of homosexual behaviour in animals." In *Homosexual behaviour in animals: An evolutionary perspective,* ed. V. Sommer and P. L. Vasey, pp. 349–64. Cambridge: Cambridge University Press.

Wald, M. S. 2001. "Same sex couple marriage: A family policy perspective." *Virginia Journal of Social Policy and the Law* 9: 291–344.

Wallace, L. 2006. "Discovering homosexuality: Cross-cultural comparison and the history of sexuality." In *Gay life and culture: A world history,* ed. R. Aldrich, pp. 249–69. London: Thames & Hudson.

Walls, N. E. 2008. Toward a multidimensional understanding of heterosexism: The changing nature of prejudice. *Journal of Homosexuality* 55(1): 20–65.

Watanabe, J. M., and B. B. Smuts. 1999. "Explaining religion without explaining it away: Trust, truth, and the evolution of cooperation in Roy A. Rappaport's 'The obvious aspects of ritual.'" *American Anthropologist* 101: 98–112.

Watanabe, T., and J. Iwata, J. 1989. *The love of the samurai: A thousand years of Japanese homosexuality.* London: Gay Men's Press.

Wellings, K., J. Wadsworth, and A. Johnson. 1994. "Sexual diversity and homosexual behavior." In *Sexual behavior in Britain: The national survey of sexual attitudes and lifestyles,* ed. K. Wellings, J. Field, A. Johnson, and J. Wadsworth, pp. 186–92. New York: Penguin.

White, M. 2000. *Leonardo: The first scientist.* New York: Saint Martin.

Whitehead, N. E. 2008. "Homosexuality and mental health problems." *NARTH: Medical Issues,* September 3. http://www.narth.com/docs/whitehead.html.

Wilford, J. N. 2005. A Mystery, Locked in Timeless Embrace. *The New York Times.* December 20. http://query.nytimes.com/gst/fullpage.html?res=9804E1DB17 30F933A15751C1A9639C8B63

Williams, C. A. 1999. *Roman homosexuality: Ideologies of masculinity in classical antiquity.* New York: Oxford University.

Winterman, D. 2008. "How 'gay' became children's insult of choice." *BBC News Magazine,* March 18. http://news.bbc.co.uk/go/pr/fr/-/1/hi/magazine/7289 390.stm.

Worthen, F. 1995. *Helping people step out of homosexuality.* 3rd ed. San Rafael, CA: New Hope Ministries.

Yamagia, J. 2006. "Playful encounters: the development of homosexual behaviour in male mountain gorillas. In *Homosexual behaviour in animals: An evolu-*

tionary perspective, ed. V. Sommer and P. L. Vasey, pp. 273–93. Cambridge: Cambridge University Press.

Zhan, S. D., and W. F. Oldenwald. 1995. "Misexpression of white (W) gene triggers male-male courtship in drosophila." *Proceeds of the National Academy of Sciences in the United States* 92: 5525–29.

Index

About the Author

Thomas (Tom) S. Serwatka is vice president and chief of staff at University of North Florida, where he has also served as the dean of graduate studies and research and an associate vice president for academic affairs. Among his various publications, Tom has coauthored chapters on LGBT issues in *Empowering Youth-At-Risk with Skills for School and Life* and in *Ethics in Education: An Anthology*. His numerous national and international presentations on social justice include "There Are No Safe Places: Gay, Lesbian, and Bisexual Youth," "Ethics, Public Schools, and Homosexuality: A Day in the Life of . . ." and "Out of the School Closet." He has served as a consultant for a host for research and development programs such as the AIDS Prevention Project of the Jacksonville Area Sexual Minority Youth Network (JASMYN), the First Coast Community AIDS Prevention Partnership, and the Florida Department of Health and Rehabilitative Services District IV U.S. Conference of Mayors AIDS Prevention Education Grant. As a community activist, Tom is currently vice chair for the board of directors of Jacksonville Area Sexual Minority Youth Network (JASMYN). He was the charter cochair for First Coast CARES (Consortium for AIDS Research, Education and Services), chair of First Coast Advisory Committee of the Northeast Florida AIDS Network and a board member for a number of other community service organizations. In addition to his work on LGBT issues, Tom's scholarship has focused on the rights of the disabled and racial minorities.